The Prakritic Diet

Dr Farah Adam Mukadam is a family physician and lactation counsellor based in Bangalore. Her first book, *Newborns and New Moms*, was a bestseller. She is a dedicated health advocate and works with NGO Focus India on its community health initiatives and medical camps.

The Prakritic Diet

Traditional Wisdom for a Bio-balanced Life

DR FARAH ADAM MUKADAM

PAN

First published 2026 by Pan
an imprint of Pan Macmillan Publishing India Private Limited
707 Kailash Building
26 K. G. Marg, New Delhi 110001
www.panmacmillan.co.in

Pan Macmillan, The Smithson, 6 Briset Street, Farringdon, London EC1M 5NR
Associated companies throughout the world
www.panmacmillan.com

ISBN 978-93-6113-221-6

1 3 5 7 9 8 6 4 2

Typeset in Calluna by R. Ajith Kumar, New Delhi
Printed and bound in India by Thomson Press India Private Limited

Disclaimer

The Author and Publisher unequivocally state that this book is intended solely for general informational and educational purposes and is not a substitute for professional medical advice, diagnosis, or treatment. The views, experiences, and recommendations presented in this book are solely those of the Author and do not reflect the opinions of the Publisher.

Readers should not disregard, delay, or substitute professional medical advice because of any information presented in this book. References to specific foods, diets, or lifestyle practices are for illustrative purposes only and should not be construed as prescriptive, diagnostic, or curative. Readers are strongly advised to consult a qualified healthcare professional before making any changes to their diet, exercise, or treatment plans.

The Author and Publisher expressly disclaim all liability for any actions, decisions, or consequences arising from the interpretation, misuse, or reliance on the content of this book.

By accessing or reading this book, readers acknowledge and accept the terms of this disclaimer. If any reader does not agree with the terms, they are advised to refrain from reading or using this book. While every effort has been made to ensure factual accuracy, the Author and Publisher shall not be held liable for any discrepancies, interpretations, or claims of reliance placed on the material contained herein.

To my father-in-law, whose love, guidance and blessings have shaped my journey in countless ways. I will carry them in my heart always.

Rest in peace.

CONTENTS

INTRODUCTION

> 'One of the first duties of the physician is to educate the masses not to take medicine'
>
> SIR WILLIAM OSLER,
> the Founder of Modern Medicine

Hi Reader!

As a family physician, I often meet patients who have undergone a full-body health check-up to advise them on their diets. With diabetes and high blood pressure (BP) running rampant in the country – lining the pockets of practically every physician and pharma company – I find myself falling back on the vague guidelines doctors usually offer: exercise more, eat less. The reality is that even we as healthcare professionals don't have complete knowledge of what to eat more of and what to avoid; which exercises to engage in, under what conditions and for how long.

Nearly every day, I come across patients who have no significant findings in their reports, yet are hassled by vague symptoms, such as their body retaining 'heat'. Another subset of patients complain of catching a cold or getting a sore throat because they ate something sour or cold. At the beginning of my career, my allopathy-trained brain shrugged off these complaints as a hangover from relying on granny-style home remedies. But then again, there was a certain uniformity in my patients' experiences.

As I dug into patient histories, it appeared curd was almost always linked with sore throats – even more often than ice cream. Pickles were also on the list of sore-throat-causing culprits. As my career progressed, the list of these so-called 'hot' and 'cold' foods kept growing longer. I could see that there was a pattern in the complaints of my patients, yet science invalidated them with nothing more than a condescending smirk and dismissive shrug.

As the years passed and I became a mother, I started getting some first-hand data. At home, my father-in-law would suggest certain foods for my kids depending on the season and weather. Another convincing piece of evidence was the time I fed my three-year-old son a banana as an evening snack. My non-medico friends discouraged me from doing so, claiming it would cause *kaff,* or phlegm. My child, who already suffered from allergic bronchitis, did indeed have mild wheezing and threw up that night, followed by a clear vomit of just phlegm. It was upsetting that my child was sick but seeing my friends' prediction come true also piqued my curiosity. So many patients and caretakers across generations were echoing each other. Were they all wrong or was contemporary science missing the bigger picture?

Western medicine backed by scientific study might be ahead in research but it lags behind in observations that have stood the test of time. It tends to seek out superfood after superfood, even though that is less a scientific category and more a genius marketing gimmick, slapped on anything exotic, overpriced or Instagram-friendly. Nutrition scientists are likely to roll their eyes at the term, since no single food can magically deliver such miracle health benefits – unless you count the miracle of rapidly emptying your wallet. Blueberries, for example, often hailed as the poster child for superfoods, are actually just moderately nutritious. No better than your average veggie.

The European Union (EU) even banned the use of the label 'superfood' in 2007 unless backed by credible scientific evidence. Translation: Unless marketers could prove the hype. Spoiler: They couldn't. Still, this dubious category thrives, especially in Western markets desperate for exotic vegetables, 'ancient grains' and 'superfruits' with mystical healing powers. Ironically, the term itself first appeared in 1949 in a Canadian newspaper to describe a muffin – yes, a muffin – which tells you everything you need to know about its scientific credibility. In the end, 'superfood' is just a fancy sticker slapped on everyday plants to make them sound like caped crusaders of nutrition, usually with a price tag to match.

I set out to find an alternative approach, one that was observational rather than theoretical. As my research progressed, I realized that Unani and Ayurveda concurred in many of their findings. The learnings and beliefs in these schools of medicine were too many to be coincidental.

Ayurveda, the traditional system of medicine that originated in India more than 3,000 years ago, is built on the idea of maintaining balance in the body, mind and spirit to achieve health. At its core are the three *doshas* – Vata, Pitta and Kapha – which are biological energies believed to govern physical and mental processes. Each person has a unique constitution, or *prakriti*, determined by the proportion of these doshas.

- **Vata** (air and space): Associated with movement, the functioning of the nervous system and creativity. When imbalanced, it can lead to anxiety, dryness or digestive issues.
- **Pitta** (fire and water): Governs metabolism, digestion and energy production. Excess Pitta may manifest as inflammation, irritability or acidity.
- **Kapha** (earth and water): Provides stability, lubrication and structure. When aggravated, it may cause sluggishness, weight gain or congestion.

Another key feature of Ayurveda is the classification of foods as 'hot' or 'cold'; not by their temperature but their energetic effect on the body.

- **Hot (*ushna*) foods** – like chili, ginger, garlic and fermented items – are said to stimulate digestion, increase metabolic heat and aggravate Pitta but balance Kapha.

- **Cold (*shita*) foods** – such as cucumber, melons, dairy and leafy greens – cool the system, soothe inflammation and are helpful for calming Pitta. However, they may aggravate Kapha or Vata if overconsumed.

Dietary prescriptions in Ayurveda are tailored to one's *doshic* balance, the season and even the time of day. The aim is always to restore harmony, prevent disease and bolster longevity through individualized nutritional and lifestyle choices.

Unani is a traditional system of healing which originated in Ancient Greece and later flourished under Arab and Persian physicians. The word 'Unani' comes from 'Ionian', meaning Greek, since it was founded on the teachings of Hippocrates and Galen, who emphasized natural causes of disease and the healing power of balance. Over the centuries, Unani medicine integrated knowledge from Indian, Persian and Arab traditions, becoming an established system of healthcare that is still practiced in India and other parts of South Asia today.

The core principle of Unani medicine is the humoural theory, which states that health depends on the balance of four body humours: blood (*dam*), phlegm (*balgham*), yellow bile (*safra*) and black bile (*sauda*). Equilibrium maintains health, while imbalance causes disease. Diagnosis and treatment focus on identifying the disruptive humour and restoring harmony through natural means.

Unani diet therapy, known as *Ilaj bil Ghiza*, is a unique non-medicinal approach wherein patients are treated and their health restored by modulating dietary habits. For instance, practitioners recommend fasting during fever episodes, or low-calorie, low-protein foods such as vegetable soups or fruits for certain ailments – such as irritable bowel syndrome (IBS) – to ease the burden on digestion. Staying true to the Unani principle, modified diets are the principal target therapy employed to treat metabolic diseases. For most chronic ailments, in fact, diet regulation serves as a preventive measure as well as therapeutic aid.

According to Unani philosophy, the nutritional value of a particular food depends on various factors, including how much of each humour it creates, what season it is and the patient's temperament. Keeping this in mind, practitioners may prescribe various types of diets: *Dawae Ghizaee* (food for nourishing a sick patient, not commonly eaten as a meal), *Ghizae Dawai* (food eaten for nourishment rather than recovery), *Kaseef Ghiza* (heavy foods), *Lateef Ghiza* (light foods), *Motadal Ghiza* (moderate foods) and many more.

Unani medicine also describes a process in which foods are broken down by the body's 'heat'. When *khamrae* (enzymes) come in contact with food, they react with it and release heat that enables digestion. This heat can be equated to the concept of *Agni* in Ayurveda – the two schools of thought have parallels galore! If you paid attention in Biology, then you know that enzymes are to our body what catalysts are to chemical reactions in the lab. Digestive enzymes like amylase and lipase speed up the chemical reactions that break down the food we consume. Everything we eat and drink is a chemical compound and thus requires a chemical breakdown.

I reiterate what I said in my first book, *Newborns and New Moms*: My aim is not to bite the hand that feeds me. I am an allopathy-trained family physician through and through. It is the lack of nutritional support and home remedies in Western medicine that prompted me to look into alternative medical branches. Despite being derived from centuries of observation, nature-aligned medical sciences continue to be seen as quackery. Even when effective, their practices are written off as a placebo effect. Over the years, I have dug into the research of these Eastern medical traditions to find insights that we can adapt to our current lifestyles in conjunction with Western treatments. This book is my effort to help you navigate the vast and often confusing landscape of nutrition, return to the innate wisdom of intuitive eating and build your health in a way that is both sensible and sustainable.

1

THE IMBALANCED, BALANCED AND BIO-BALANCED DIET

While Eastern medical traditions focus on balance, modern life appears to be spiralling in the opposite direction. In an age of cutting-edge medicine, we are paradoxically plagued by vague 'lifestyle diseases' that no pill seems to cure: metabolic syndrome, unexplained fatigue, prediabetes, obesity, autoimmune disease and chronic inflammation, among others. Instead of clarity, there is an epidemic of excess information. We wake to every influencer and brand ambassador prescribing a new 'super drink' to gulp first thing in the morning. Lemon juice with honey? Apple cider vinegar? Holy spring water with chia seeds that have been soaking overnight? The confusion is endless, fuelled by food lobbies that would rather keep us buying than informed.

Meanwhile, 'lifestyle modification' has become the most casually scribbled line on a doctor's prescription pad, even as there is no consensus on what that actually entails. Just two decades ago, walking was dismissed as the exercise of the elderly; now it's glorified by smartwatches counting our every step. Health has become a scoreboard and our food choices are dictated by marketing labels and algorithms. Meal planning has been outsourced to influencers, internet quacks, fad diet prophets and gym trainers who care more about protein shake sales than our actual well-being. Sorry if you are engaged in one of these occupations but ... genuinely, I'm not sorry. Despite medical advancements, we are the unhealthiest generation in history when it comes to preventable lifestyle illnesses and the noise around health has only made us more lost.

If you ever wondered why nutrition and health guidelines feel suspiciously watered down, just follow the money. The American Diabetes Association (ADA) – the very body advising millions on diabetes and diet – takes money from consumer-product companies like Splenda that benefit when certain foods are viewed as benign or even healthy.[1] Mars Inc. (via Wrigley) has also partnered with the ADA's Dental Health Foundation for the 'Healthier Smiles' grants to promote oral health.[2] Let me break this down for you. Mars is a candy company. Its products include Mars, M&Ms, Snickers and Bounty to name a few – sticky, caramelly, peanuty, coconuty chocolate bars that are a big NO for oral health. Amirite? But the cunning lies in how the antidote to poor oral health is also their product – sugar-free Wrigley's chewing gum!

Organizations like the American College of Obstetricians & Gynecologists and breast cancer societies have also received funding or sponsorship from formula companies, pharmaceutical firms, alcohol or processed food sectors (especially via pink-ribbon campaigns), muddying advocacy messages.[3,4]

In a study of scientific societies in Spain active in childhood nutrition and obesity prevention between 2017–18, Nestlé was identified as sponsoring about 36 per cent of such foundations. This revelation is egregious given the highly processed, nutritionally deficient products that form the bulk of Nestlé's catalogue and the company's history of neglecting public health.[5]

Starting in the 1960s, Nestlé aggressively marketed infant formula across Africa, Asia and Latin America, portraying breastfeeding – the gold standard for infant nutrition – as outdated, unsafe or insufficient for the modern baby. Nestlé saleswomen dressed in crisp white nurse uniforms visited new mothers in hospitals, handing out free formula that lasted just long enough to reduce their natural breast milk supply, creating dependency. Families, unable to afford the expensive formula and often lacking clean water, diluted it. This led to malnutrition, diarrhoea and, in many cases, infant deaths.[6] The scandal sparked global outrage, boycotts and partial rollbacks but Nestlé continues to dominate the infant formula and baby food market via Gerber.

Nestlé has since been accused of selling baby cereals in lower-income countries with far more sugar than in wealthier markets.[7,8] Premade purees for infants, even without the additional sugar, pave the way for future obesity.[9] Calorie-dense, nutrient-poor foods like Maggi noodles, chocolate bars and other easy-to-eat snacks target children, driving obesity, poor diet quality and an early preference for sweets. These highly processed convenience products are part of the global nutrition transition away from whole foods. The company's so-called health drinks, Nesquik and Milo, have been criticized for confusing buyers about their health value. In fact, a Nesquik campaign guaranteeing a 'great start to the day' was banned in some jurisdictions for misleading consumers. Nestlé's strategy is a textbook example of marketing overriding public health. And let me remind you, they are the gatekeepers of childhood nutrition and obesity prevention.

It's a page from the old tobacco industry playbook – the companies most at fault for disease also bankroll the bodies 'educating' the public.[10] Food and pharma lobbies make the mess, sell the fix and kick our asses on their way out.

The Imbalanced Diet

Let me pause here to clarify that a diet consists of what we eat – the presence of food rather than its absence. In contrast to this, over the 1970s and 80s, there emerged extremely imbalanced diets condemning our stomachs for wanting food, our tongues for craving flavour and our bodies for demanding energy (calories, in internet-speak).

I'll start with one of the most 'extra' diets that came onto the stage in the 1980s: the extreme gas-forming cabbage soup diet. The proponents of this diet claimed you could lose around 4–5 kilograms of weight in a week. Miraculous and too good to be true, isn't it? And true it wasn't.

A diet that consists almost entirely of cabbage soup deprives our body of protein while overloading it with sodium. One of the reasons why this is the rock bottom of all diets is because of how restrictive it is. I distinctly remember, as a third grader, being fascinated as we were introduced to energy-providing carbohydrates, scurvy-preventing vitamins and building block proteins. Somehow, even today, eight-year-olds have more knowledge about eating well than a large chunk of confused adults.

Despite these obvious weaknesses, did the cabbage soup diet do anyone any good?

Yes, if our definition of good is determined purely by the weighing scale. This diet appeared to work because it was so high in fibre. The fibre would make one feel full initially and draw more water into the intestine. Simple physics at play here. But limiting one's food intake in this way had a long list of disadvantages.

The way one lost weight while on this diet was by shedding both water weight and muscle mass. Our bodies are 70 per cent water. Since this diet provided the body with such limited calories, the carbohydrate stores in the muscle – known as glycogen – were used to supplement energy. Glycogen binds to water and when your reserves are spent because you are on a low-carb diet, this water weight is what is first lost. A noteworthy fact is that glycogen is replenished each day (unlike our fat stores) and is the first to be spent in times of starvation. And starve one did on the soup diet! The worst part is that the diet resulted in muscle loss. Remember, there is barely any protein in this diet. As a result, the body essentially eats up its own muscles to provide proteins to the undernourished body.

The proponents of the cabbage diet said that it should be followed only for a week or two. Please be warned, any short-term weight loss programme which promises instant results is steering you towards lowered metabolism and this change is irreversible more often than not. The fat loss from this diet is minimal. But the hangry feeling? Oh, so inevitable!

When a person is in good health they are brimming with vitality. Restricting yourself to eating only cabbage soup has the opposite effect. A person observing this diet will be low on energy and irritable. If you opt for this bizarre diet for a function or even your wedding, the outcome will not be what you want. Your skin will lack lustre, your face will lose its glow and your mood will be at grumpiness-max!

A decade before the cabbage diet, the Atkins diet was all the rage. Famous cardiologist Robert Atkins designed this diet based on the assumption that carbohydrates were the sole cause of health and heart problems. It was similar to a present-day fad, the keto diet. Across three stages, the extremely low-carb Atkins diet eliminated all the 'unhealthy' carbs from one's plate to achieve weight loss. For the Western world, this meant maida (refined flour) products had to be cut out. In India, the most popular carbs happened to be rice, roti, idli and dosa.

The issues with this diet were manifold.

First off, our brains are designed to use glucose from carbohydrates as the first choice of fuel. So, the 'hanger' (anger caused by hunger) of the subject was through the roof from lack of glucose.

Second, even though the subject consumed proteins and fats (a big win for the cravings), an entire subgroup of foods was eliminated, depriving them of vitamins and minerals. In search of itty-bitty waists, we lay to waste our itty-bitty nutrients – the micros.

The heavy protein load was too much for the kidneys to take. The long-term effects of the Atkins diet were constipation (we want daily bowel movement, please!), kidney stones, irritability, low productivity and fatigue, thanks to the lack of carbs. Some patients even developed bone weakness, or osteoporosis.

I won't say this diet was absolute rubbish like the cabbage soup one. There were some advantages: it helped kickstart weight loss (though temporarily) and reduced total cholesterol and triglycerides, which was great for some patients. However, following restrictive diets and omitting entire food groups irreversibly lowers metabolism. Extreme weight loss followed by anxiety about regaining weight once normal food habits resume results in a yo-yo effect, so to speak. And once you are on that yo-yo, your weight loss definitely goes slow-slow.

Over the years, many other restrictive diets have surfaced. The polyphenol diet recommended eating mostly fruits and veggies, skipping grains and pulses. This can lead to a whole host of kidney issues, as discussed later in this book. Then an era was devoted to removing every molecule of fat from our diets. Then came the love for protein with one shunned loner – gluten. Now we are obsessed with keto just like our on-screen role models.

Still, some people are starting to realize the fallacy of these many experiments. We humans are modern-day lab rats in more ways than we think. Frequently and willingly, we give in to the latest diet trends, providing scientists with data on the benefits – and more often, the pitfalls – of such diets.

We are very consenting guinea pigs, if you will.

Eating Well: Local or Global?

There are so many foods these days that are leaving their hometowns only to find themselves all the way across the world on the plates of the calorie-conscious gym rats or those just trying to keep up with the pace of superfood discoveries. The fad that riles me up the most is quinoa. Native to the Andes mountains of South America, the global discovery of this food – super-rich in vitamin C and E – by the health-conscious has contributed to the malnutrition epidemic in Peru. Once a Peruvian staple, quinoa is now the government's cash cow as it exports the entire crop. As global demand continues to climb, quinoa prices have skyrocketed, spiking up to three times within a few years, pushing it further out of reach for many local families. And what are the locals who grow this highly nutritious grain left with? Cheap, greasy take-out – the perfect recipe for malnutrition.[11]

Let's now look at the Mediterranean region. Corruption in the olive oil export industry has been an ongoing issue. In his book *Extra Virginity*, investigative journalist Tom Mueller exposed unscrupulousness in the global olive oil trade. He revealed how a large share of the oil sold as 'extra virgin' is in fact diluted with lower-grade refined oils or produced from substandard olives, misleading consumers and undercutting honest producers. Systematic corruption – involving large-scale adulteration with cheap seed oils, mislabelling and powerful trade cartels – intensified in the late twentieth century, especially in the last two decades. This period saw globalization of olive oil markets, weak enforcement of quality standards and organized crime networks exploiting high profits. The result is a marketplace where profit often outweighs purity, tradition and consumer trust.

If the malnourishment of the Peruvian children and scandalous olive oil export industry aren't enough, let me take you on another trip across the Atlantic to Mexico – the land of avocados.

Despite being one of the most expensive fruits, the

craze for avocado is far from over. This pricey cash crop has contributed to a rise in organized crime in Mexico. A report published in 2019 by global risk intelligence firm Maplecroft claimed that avocado could be the next 'conflict commodity': 'From cultivation through to transportation, violence and corruption now pervade Mexico's avocado supply chain.'[12]

The report went on to say that the perpetrators steal about four truckloads of avocado a day and have started to compete with local farmers in cultivating this fruit. Let alone the humble farmer, even shipping and packaging facilities are not safe from extortion. While some farmers have picked up arms to protect their avocado businesses, others rely on private security forces. Yet neither violence nor saturation of the cultivators all over Mexico has curbed the insatiable demand for avocado worldwide – and its profitability.

And the issue is far-reaching. While this green gold is at the heart of Mexican exports, the conversion of Portugal into an avocado exporter is nothing short of criminal. The avocado plant is a thirsty one and Portugal is a country that faces drought-like conditions. You can live without your avocado toast but the Portuguese can't live without water.[13,14]

It's become a trend to raise crops in unnatural habitats to feed the hungry 'good-fat-conscious' health fiends. But lives are being ruined and lost to fulfil this bottomless appetite for quinoa, kale, avocado and many other fad foods. God knows which alleged superfood will be in vogue by the time this book gets published. I'm spotlighting the hidden backstories behind today's 'superfoods' to show how our global food obsessions drive damaging trends. I urge you to rethink your food choices. As the consumers, we create demand. But we must refuse to become parasites. The shift begins with us. Allow distant communities to keep their native grains. And closer to home, create space on your plate for amazing local foods and support our farmers.

While we sit in the comfort of our homes and buy quinoa, olive oil and avocados off our grocery apps, we need to take a step back and look at the bigger picture. At what cost are we craving non-regional, out-of-season foods?

Today's Balanced Diet

I once saw a video asking viewers to eat packets and packets of green leafy vegetables. No context, no background. Simply claiming that one needs to consume fibre as per the recommended daily allowance (RDA) guidelines and this giant packet of greens was the solution to all health- and weight-related woes.

Think back to those old 2D cartoons: Why does Popeye eat spinach all the time? Your instant reply might be that spinach is one of the best sources of iron. More iron means more strength – it's that simple, isn't it? No, not really. One of the reasons why spinach is considered a storehouse of iron is because an oft-quoted study erroneously claimed that the iron content was ten times the actual number. A wrongly placed decimal point helped perpetuate this myth.[15]

Today, one single video can spread just as widely and be taken as gospel truth if it taps into people's need to carefully observe the RDA guidelines. This is the brand of hyper-optimization of diets that runs rampant on social media. But remember, no one diet fits all. I will keep bringing up this point in relevant contexts throughout the book.

This brings me to the question: How practical and logical is it to have a balanced, eat-the-rainbow plate for every meal on a daily basis?

Not at all logical. When you have a fever, you tend to lose your appetite and rest more so that your body can recruit its blood cells for recovery rather than waste resources digesting a meal. While winters are for eating more fat- and carb-rich foods, our body functions best in the summer on a light, nourishing diet with abundant sources of fluid like cucumber and watermelon.

The Bio-balanced Diet

> 'Let food be thy medicine and medicine be thy food'
>
> HIPPOCRATES

Food is not just nutrition and our digestive system is more than a hollow tube from mouth to anus. It follows principles of physics, chemistry and biology.

The physics is the change in blood flow to different

parts of the gut by the mere thought and smell of food; the pushing movement of the gut that propels food forward without being too dependent on gravity. The chemistry is the reserve of enzymes and hormones that regulate digestion by giving feedback to the preceding and succeeding enzymes. The biology is the feedback the mouth, stomach and intestine give to the brain during eating and digestion. The brain then guides you to a point of satiety.

Modern science has recently warmed up to the idea of taste playing a role in digestion. It has been discovered that our tongue is not the only body part that can taste. We have taste receptors right from the tip of the tongue all the way down to our intestines. The distribution of taste receptors suggests that the gut is capable of sensing and responding to the chemical composition of ingested food far beyond the initial tasting.

These taste receptors are part of a complex system that helps the body sense and respond to different types of nutrients and chemical compounds in the ingested food. Taste receptors in the gut contribute to nutrient sensing and help the body distinguish between varied kinds of food. This nutrient sensing is involved in the regulation of many digestive functions, such as insulin release, appetite control and energy metabolism.

Various types of taste receptors are sensitive to specific compounds. For instance, sweet taste receptors in the intestines trigger the release of hormones that stimulate the absorption of glucose. The gut is connected to the brain through the gut-brain axis and taste receptors in the gut are involved in signalling this axis. Signals from gut taste receptors influence sensations of hunger and satiety and impact our overall eating behaviour. Dysregulation of gut taste receptors has been implicated in health conditions like obesity and metabolic disorders.

Ayurveda points to a driving force, Agni, that helps digestion. Agni, literally meaning 'fire', refers to the increase in blood supply to different parts of the intestine as soon as the digested slurry of food – also called chyme – reaches there. The *Vipaka* – or aftertaste – is a product of the action of the digestive Agni on the foods we eat. Vipaka also affects the taste receptors in the entirety of the gut and controls subsequent processes in food digestion. The importance Ayurveda gave to taste is now emerging in food science with the discovery of pungent receptors in the human gut. These receptors help control food movement and digestion. In fact, the conversion from bitter to pungent taste as per the Vipaka theory has now been uncovered by science as well.[16]

Research shows that bitter-tasting food has the capacity to rejuvenate gut function. For example, our favourite morning drink of lemon in water derives its benefits from the bitter rind (peel) of the fruit. Lemon, strongly aromatic and slightly bitter, has been variously used both in the West and East as a digestive tonic, in decoctions and alcoholic extracts. In addition to being a digestive, it has traditionally been employed as an anti-spasmodic and carminative (gas-releasing) agent. The sour taste of lemon drives a reflexive cheek-puckering, eye-squinting reaction and increases salivation to wash away the acidic taste from the mouth. When the saliva floods our mouth, a signal is sent to the brain to ready the rest of the digestive tract with enzymes and juices for digestion.

The presence of these non-tasting bitter receptors through the digestive system activates and promotes the release of a local hormone in the gut called cholecystokinin (CCK). This in turn activates the release of enzymes from the pancreas and bile salts from the liver for digesting fats and carbohydrates. These receptors also regulate the movement of food in the gut, boost gastric acid secretion, slow down the emptying of food from the stomach and leave us satiated. Bitter receptor activation aims at reducing the absorption of bitter compounds and maximizing the absorption of complex carbohydrates, essential fatty acids and fat-soluble vitamins.

The major impact of bitter tasting foods on digestion is improved blood circulation in the abdominal organs. This reaction is called hyperaemia. A person suffering from piles (haemorrhoids) or intestinal ulcers who ingests something bitter will therefore make the condition worse because of this post-digestive effect. Following digestion, bitter changes to pungent, resulting in a burning sensation, bleeding and inflammation as the digested food reaches the rectum and anus.

Ayurveda associates sourness with a post-digestive effect that stimulates digestion. This is known as Amla

Vipaka – taken from amla, the Indian gooseberry and one of the sourest foods of all. Modern science agrees that the acids present in sour foods influence gastric acid secretion and digestive enzyme activity. Heating and stimulating effects are attributed to pungent tastes called *Katu* Vipaka. Scientifically, compounds responsible for pungency, such as capsaicin, activate thermoreceptors and influence metabolic rate.

As allopathy catches on to the wisdom of Unani and Ayurvedic medicine, a hypothesis emerges. Bitter food can be used to reduce the gastric emptying rate (allowing gastric secretions to act on foods for a longer period) and enhance the post-gastric digestion of fats and complex carbohydrates. Clinical data also points to anti-dyspeptic (anti-indigestion) activity produced by the examined bitter-tasting plants.[17]

Some gut ailments, such as IBS, can be addressed using the essential oil of peppermint and peppermint tea or water. These reduce the pressure build-up in the walls of the colon, relieve spasming and facilitate emptying of the bowel. Bitter compounds slow down food transit through the intestine and promote adequate absorption of nutrients from the macros, eliminating bloating. IBS is predominant in the Vata dosha (gas-forming imbalance) and medicines such peppermint essential oil and *shahjeera* (caraway seeds) help promote removal of gas by reducing the cramping of the bowel and free the patient from bloating.

The scientific mind might reason that these taste

receptors are in fact chemical sensors placed all over your gut. It follows that these functions are just your receptors reacting to the corresponding molecules. I thought the same at first. But over time, I have been proven wrong. As an example, consider the zero-calorie artificial sweetener saccharin. It is marketed as a sugar alternative that can help you control your diabetes – and your waistline. That couldn't be further from the truth.

The sweet taste of saccharin on your tongue tells the pancreas to secrete insulin. Even though it contains no glucose, your body reacts to the mere taste of sweetness in the same way as it would to a load of glucose. This insulin spike is a response to an empty signal – the artificial sweetener. Insulin is responsible for moving glucose into cells. When you consume artificially sweetened food, you end up with high levels of insulin but no glucose for the body to break down. This maladaptive response results in insulin resistance, the starting point of a cascade of metabolic diseases such as diabetes and heart disease.

In short, taste matters.

The Transparent Diet

With every season, Mother Earth offers us something different. In the winter, we crave food that is fatty and high in sugar. It is no surprise that most Indian festivals arrive with the cold, perfect for our body to enjoy all the ghee-laden goodies. Madhura, or sweetness, is one of the *rasas* (tastes) found naturally – not just in conventional desserts but carbohydrate-rich grains and fruits too.

Rather than your watch calculating calories and steps, I recommend letting your tastebuds guide the way to what you and your body desire and deserve.

To strike that physical, mental and emotional equilibrium, we need to be balanced in the qualities we consume. Each taste signifies its place in our diet and even tells us how the substance will affect our bodies, which ultimately will govern our state of mind.

The oldest taste in evolutionary history is that of sourness. Right from the time when our ancestors lived in the oceans and were yet to move to land, the sour taste diffused into the surrounding water warned them of danger.[18] The acidity indicated less oxygen and more carbon dioxide, prompting them to move away. Till date, most mammals and birds have a strong sense of the acidic – or sour – taste.

As we evolved, our bodies learnt that this acidity is not dangerous to consume. Quite the contrary, it is super beneficial for us and unhealthy to avoid. Unfortunately, millions of years ago, the gene for producing vitamin C in our bodies underwent a mutation and lost its functionality. Vitamin C happens to be an acid and thus has a sour taste. Our ancestors intuitively sought out the taste to ensure their well-being and protection from the deficiency disease scurvy.

As life went from sea-dwelling to land-dwelling, from monkey to man, many animals lost their sense of certain tastes. For instance, cats are not capable of discerning sweetness. However, research conducted in 2022 led to the discovery that there is not a single species of animal (vertebrate) that cannot taste sourness.[19] This is the genetic result of evolutionary necessity.

Other tastes are linked to the nutritional composition of food, too. Salty and sweet flavours attract us with the promise of sodium and glucose. Bitterness warns us against foods which could be potentially toxic. Umami – though not defined in Ayurveda and Unani – is your staple savoury taste. It indicates richness in proteins that are essential for our growth and maintenance.

Sweet foods are heavy and stabilizing, moist and nourishing. Their overall after-effect on digestion is cooling and calming. In Ayurvedic medicine, an emphasis on the sweet taste is recommended for those who are weak or emaciated, or the young and elderly. However, sweet taste in excess is kapha producing. Recent research has identified that diabetics have a higher likelihood of chronic lung disease with excess phlegm production. The study pointed out that, irrespective of age and smoking habits, long-term mucus production is one of the under-reported symptoms of diabetes.[20] This is in accordance with our traditional medical knowledge that excess madhura rasa (sweet) results in increased kapha (in this context, mucus). It is important to note that kapha is not merely mucus or phlegm, as translated from Sanskrit. In the next chapter I go into the fundamentals of the Kapha dosha, so let's put that on hold for now.

Overindulging in the sweet taste – typically carbohydrate-rich food – can result in sluggishness and lethargy; heaviness and weight gain; an excess of mucus and slow digestion. High sugar intake can suppress the immune system, too. The increased level of sugar has the potential to inhibit the work of white blood cells, which help ward off infection. Poor immunity and delayed wound healing are among the most profound effects of diabetes. Remember, everything can be a poison (even love) – it just depends on the dose.

Balance According to Unani

Unani has a concept called *Mizaj*, or the temperament of food. Mizaj plays a crucial role in understanding the inherent properties of various substances, including food. These temperaments are believed to have an impact on the balance of the entire body. The most basic tenet of Unani is '*Hifzus Sehah*' – medicine is the preservation of health and restoring it when it gets lost.

According to Unani principles, maintaining a balance between the humours (more on humours in the next chapter) is essential for health and consuming foods with the right Mizaj can help achieve this balance.

Here's an overview of the temperaments of food in Unani medicine:

1. **Hot *(Har)*:** Foods with a hot temperament increase heat in the body. They are recommended for people with a cold temperament or those who need to balance excess cold in their bodies.
2. **Cold *(Barid)*:** These foods have a cooling effect on the body. Suggested for individuals with a hot

temperament or those who need to balance excess heat.

3. **Wet (*Rutubat*):** These foods provide moisture and are recommended for individuals with a dry temperament.
4. **Dry (*Yabis*):** In the same vein, dry temperament foods are believed to have a drying effect on the body. They are suggested for individuals with excessive moisture.

The principle of *Mizaj Tadawi* describes the therapeutic balancing of different tastes to maintain health. A parallel in Ayurveda would be the rasas. Since I uncovered the link between the nature of food and tastes through studying Unani, I will be exploring this topic from that lens. However, aside from the naming of the tastes, there is very little difference between the two pedagogies. The key principle is to achieve balance among the four temperaments: hot, cold, wet and dry. This balance is often achieved by judiciously combining different tastes in the diet. For example, a meal may include a combination of sweet and sour tastes to balance coldness and moisture. The quintessential Indian gravy base of onion and tomatoes fulfils this criterion.

The art of balancing tastes in traditional medicine is tailored to individual constitutions. Practitioners carefully select foods and spices to achieve a harmonious equilibrium. This personalized approach can be adopted in our daily lives as well. Each taste, with its unique combination of nature, quality and effect, plays a distinctive role in balancing the body's temperaments and promoting overall health.

In the next two chapters I will elaborate on different body temperaments and how to develop your intuition when it comes to food. In the subsequent chapters, I'll dive into the bio-nature (*taseer*) of various foods – whether they are hot or cold; when and how to consume them while accounting for your natural temperament and temperament imbalances throughout the year due to illness or environmental influences.

Unani offers us a very simple guide that helps us understand the taste (*zaika*) and taseer of food. You may refer to it while learning to adopt the intuitive method of eating.

1. Sweet Taste (Rasa-e-Mulavi)

- **Effect/Tabe'a:** Nutritive (Tadawi)
- Sweet taste is cold, heavy and nutritive. Characterized by its heaviness, the sweet taste imparts a sense of fullness and substantiality. Sweet foods are great sources of proteins, fats and carbs.
- The sweet taste contributes significantly to the nourishment and vitality of the body. It is recommended in conditions marked by excess heat or dryness, where it aids in restoring balance through coolness and moisture.
- Dates are recommended for individuals with excess heat or dryness. Their heavy and nutritive nature

provides nourishment and strength, restoring balance through coolness and moisture.

2. *Sour Taste (Rasa-e-Hamid)*

- **Effect/Tabe'a:** Refrigerant (Muhallil)
- Sour taste is cold and moist. Associated with moisture, the sour taste contributes to hydration and is recommended for those with a dry temperament.
- Known for its refrigerant properties (Muhallil), the sour taste helps reduce body heat. It is recommended in conditions where cooling and moisture need to be balanced.
- Lemon, with its sour taste, is suitable for those with excess heat. The sourness has both a cooling effect and moist quality, acting as a refrigerant to reduce body heat.

3. *Salty Taste (Rasa-e-Milh)*

- **Effect/Tabe'a:** Lubricant (Mulheq)
- Salty taste is hot and moist. With its moisture-attracting quality, this taste is hydrating and recommended for those with a dry temperament, as it helps restore moisture balance.
- The salty taste acts as a lubricant (Mulheq), facilitating smoother movement of bodily fluids.
- Sea salt has these moisture-trapping and lubricative qualities, making it suitable for those with a dry temperament. It facilitates smoother movement of bodily fluids.

4. Bitter Taste (Rasa-e-Murr)

- **Effect/Tabe'a:** Detoxicant (Tanzil)
- Alongside its cold nature, the bitter taste is associated with dryness and addresses conditions marked by an excess of moisture in the body.
- The bitter taste is designated as a Tanzil (detoxicant). In Unani medicine, it is recommended for individuals exhibiting a hot or moist temperament. With its unique combination of cold nature, dry quality and detoxicant effect, the bitter taste plays a crucial role in restoring balance in conditions associated with heat and excess moisture within the body.
- Bitter gourd reduces sugar spikes and helps detoxify the body, aiding in the elimination of excess moisture and toxins.

5. Pungent Taste (Rasa-e-Har)

- **Effect/Tabe'a:** Stimulant (Mudir)
- Pungent taste is hot and dry. With its light quality, the pungent taste invigorates and awakens. This makes it beneficial for those with an excess of heaviness.
- Known for its stimulant properties, the pungent taste promotes improved digestion and circulation. It is recommended when increased warmth and lightness are required.
- The pungent taste of chili pepper provides warmth and stimulation. It is recommended for those with excess coldness since it promotes improved digestion and circulation.

6. Astringent Taste (Rasa-e-Kasila)

- **Effect/Tabe'a:** Binding (Muhallil)
- Associated with dryness, the astringent taste aids in reducing excess moisture in the body. This quality is especially useful for those with a hot and moist temperament.
- The astringent taste is known for its binding properties and contributes to the toning and tightening of tissues. It is recommended for individuals who are looking to reduce excess moisture and promote tissue firmness.
- Pomegranate, with its astringent taste, is recommended for individuals with excess heat. Its cold and dry nature, along with the binding effect it has, helps tone and tighten tissues.

Balance According to Ayurveda

The three doshas – Vata, Pitta and Kapha – are fundamental elements or energies that are central to the principles of Ayurveda. These doshas are characterized as dynamic forces that govern a person's physiological and psychological functions. Ayurvedic treatments and recommendations aim to restore balance to the doshas and address specific health concerns based on an individual's constitution and current imbalances. *Prakruti* is the term used to describe one's inherent constitution, while *Vikruti* refers to one's current state of health.

1. Prakruti

Prakruti is an individual's natural, genetic and constitutional makeup. It is the unique combination of the three fundamental bio-energies or doshas present at the time of birth, which influence one's physical and psychological traits, tendencies and susceptibilities. Due to a lack of suitable vocabulary in contemporary Western medicine, you will find me going back to the term 'dosha' throughout my book. Bio-energy is the closest term. Similarly, there is no exact equivalent in traditional Chinese medicine (TCM), since both Western medicine and TCM have different diagnostic and treatment paradigms.

However, in TCM, there exists a similar concept of an individual's inherent balance of energies – Yin–yang. Yin signifies the feminine nurturing energy while Yang is the masculine provider. Both coexist and need to be in balance for the body to be at its optimal best. Mizaj, as understood in Unani medicine, is also somewhat analogous to Prakruti.

2. Vikruti

Vikruti represents an individual's current state of health, including any imbalances in their doshas. It reflects deviations from their natural Prakruti due to changing factors like diet, lifestyle, environment and stress. In TCM, the practice of *Zheng*, or pattern diagnosis, is somewhat analogous to Vikruti. In Unani medicine, *Su-*

e-Mizaj refers to an individual's state of Mizaj, which can become imbalanced due to external factors. This concept is akin to Vikruti in Ayurveda.

Assessing Prakruti and Achieving Balance

Ayurveda is a holistic system of medicine that considers an individual's unique constitution and imbalances when recommending treatments. Assessing Prakruti and Vikruti helps practitioners provide personalized and effective healthcare. The aim is to maintain the patient's natural constitution, or Prakruti, by harmonizing the doshas through diet, lifestyle changes and therapeutic approaches.

To assess Prakruti, Ayurvedic practitioners use a combination of methods, including physical examination, pulse diagnosis and detailed questioning about the patient's physical, mental and emotional tendencies. There are also Ayurvedic questionnaires and assessments that can help identify an individual's Prakruti.

To make things easier for you, I have collated two questionnaires. The first will assess your original body type (Prakruti) and the second will study disturbances in your bio-energy to deduce your Vikruti. These forms are just to give you an idea of what to focus on when we start to decode the nature of food and the environment in subsequent chapters.

Ayurvedic Prakruti Self-Assessment Form

You can go through this questionnaire and assign points based on your lifelong tendencies.

Physical Attributes

1. **Body Build**
   - Slender (BMI below 18.5): 0 points
   - Moderate (BMI between 18.5 and 24.9): 1 point
   - Sturdy (BMI 25 or above): 2 points

You can calculate your BMI using this formula: BMI = weight (in kg)/height (in metres) squared

2. **Hair Texture**
   - Fine or thin: 0 points
   - Moderate: 1 point
   - Thick or wavy: 2 points

3. **Skin Texture**
   - Sensitive, dry: 0 points
   - Moderate: 1 point
   - Thick, oily: 2 points

Mental and Emotional Attributes

4. **Mental Tendencies**
   - Creative, imaginative: 0 points
   - Analytical, intellectual: 1 point
   - Methodical, practical: 2 points

5. **Emotional Tendencies**
   - Anxious, restless: 0 points
   - Irritable, competitive: 1 point
   - Calm, patient: 2 points

Digestive Traits

6. **Appetite**
   - Irregular or variable: 0 points
   - Strong, but can skip meals: 1 point
   - Consistent and hearty: 2 points

7. **Digestion**
   - Variable, prone to gas: 0 points
   - Strong, prone to acidity: 1 point
   - Slow but steady: 2 points

Tolerance to Climate

8. **Climate Preferences**
   - Prefers warmth, dislikes cold: 0 points
   - Tolerates both: 1 point
   - Prefers cold, dislikes heat: 2 points

Final Scoring

Add up the points from each section to determine your predominant Prakruti:

- 0-5 points: Predominantly Vata
- 6-10 points: Predominantly Pitta
- 11-14 points: Predominantly Kapha

This self-assessment is a simplified indication of your predominant Prakruti. Prakruti assessment is best conducted by a trained Ayurvedic practitioner through a comprehensive examination.

Ayurvedic Vikruti Self-Assessment Form

Determining your current doshic imbalance through a self-assessment can provide some insight into your present state of health based on Ayurvedic principles. Here's a simplified form that uses a point system to assess your Vikruti.

Assign points based on the severity and frequency of your current physical symptoms.

Current Physical Symptoms

1. **Digestive Symptoms**
   - Gas, bloating, irregular bowel movements: 0 points
   - Occasional acidity or indigestion: 1 point
   - Frequent indigestion, heartburn or constipation: 2 points

2. **Skin Symptoms**
   - Occasional dryness or minor skin issues: 0 points
   - Moderate skin issues (rashes, acne, etc.): 1 point
   - Chronic or severe skin issues: 2 points

3. **Energy Levels**
   - Consistently high energy: 0 points
   - Some fluctuations in energy: 1 point

- Low energy or chronic fatigue: 2 points

Mental and Emotional Symptoms

4. **Stress and Anxiety**
    - Occasional stress or anxiety: 0 points
    - Moderate stress or anxiety: 1 point
    - Chronic/severe stress or anxiety: 2 points

5. **Irritability**
    - Occasional irritability: 0 points
    - Moderate irritability: 1 point
    - Frequent irritability or anger: 2 points

6. **Mood Swings**
    - Occasional mood swings: 0 points
    - Moderate mood swings: 1 point
    - Frequent or severe mood swings: 2 points

Sleep Patterns

7. **Sleep Quality**
    - Restful and sound sleep: 0 points
    - Occasional sleep disturbances: 1 point
    - Frequent sleep disturbances or insomnia: 2 points

Dietary and Lifestyle Habits

8. **Diet**
    - Balanced and mindful eating: 0 points
    - Occasional unhealthy eating habits: 1 point
    - Consistently poor dietary choices: 2 points

Final Scoring

Add up the points from each section to determine your current Vikruti:

- 0-5 points: Predominantly Balanced
- 6-10 points: Predominantly Vata Imbalance
- 11-14 points: Predominantly Pitta Imbalance
- 15-20 points: Predominantly Kapha Imbalance

With your scores before you, we stand at the edge of a forgotten truth – one that Western medicine has ignored, reducing the extraordinary symphony of our bodies to cold, inanimate cells. In its drive for exactness, Western science has disregarded the miracle within, seeing the heart as nothing but a pump, the brain as nothing but a computer and our cells as nothing but static building blocks. In the next chapter I shall bridge the gap between sixth century BC physicians Sushruta and Charaka and Anthony Fauci circa 2025.

2

THE REDUCED HUMAN

The Cell Theory

Modern science has reduced us humans to a collection of cells. Just as social media continues to overwhelm our lives, diluting people to mere images and aesthetics, science has long portrayed humans as nothing more than a biological progression from monkey to man. You see, there's reductionism everywhere.

The reductive approach in Western medicine – breaking the body into cells, organs and molecular pathways – has been crucial for scientific progress, enabling targeted therapy, precise diagnostics, surgical innovation and evidence-based intervention. By isolating specific mechanisms, scientists have developed cancer drugs, insulin therapy, organ transplants and advanced imaging techniques, dramatically extending life. Yet, this focus on parts rather than the whole sometimes backfires; it can fail to account for the body's self-regulatory systems, psychosocial factors and interconnected physiology, leading to treatments that address symptoms but not root causes.

In fact, that is one of the biggest pitfalls of modern medicine: there are no cures, only 'treatments' which go on indefinitely more often than not. This limiting viewpoint has led scientists and doctors to wander further and further away from the fine art of clinical observation. They have inadvertently turned a blind eye to the body's innate will to heal itself. The reductive lens, while indispensable, risks overlooking the living complexity it seeks to heal.

Let me simplify this. My mother-in-law's BP recently shot up. She is quite averse to seeking medical help, so it took some effort and emotional blackmail to get her to my hospital to investigate the issue. On the way, I spoke to a few of my colleagues who specialize in internal medicine, endocrinology and cardiology. The internist asked me to run kidney function tests. That's it. The endocrinologist insisted my mother-in-law get blood work done to rule out something called Conn's syndrome. The cardiologist asked for an ECG and Echocardiogram.

All three of them are fantastic doctors. Yet they all focused on what they always focus on: their pet organ system. Their rigorous but super-specialized clinical acumen has been trained to zero in on a fraction of the full story. The more we super-specialize as physicians and surgeons, the less we tend to focus on the overall human body. That is the result of reductionism in modern science.

Reductionism often fosters a divide between different branches of medicine. Specialists focusing on specific organs or systems might miss crucial connections that could be vital for diagnosis and treatment. A more interdisciplinary approach, considering the whole body and mind, is necessary to provide comprehensive healthcare.

Another consequence of reductionism is the tendency to oversimplify the human body and its intricate workings. By isolating individual components, such as genes or molecules, it often disregards the holistic nature of health. Human beings are not simply a sum total of individual parts. Rather, our bodies are complex systems wherein all the elements are in conversation in subtle yet profound ways.

Like every single ecosystem in nature, the human body needs to maintain a delicate balance. It needs to be seen not just under a microscope but through the doctor's eyes, ears, intuition and experience. Reductionism is the mother of gross oversight of the environmental, social and psychological factors that significantly impact physical health. A disease might have genetic origins, but it is also influenced by the patient's lifestyle, stress, socio-economic status and cultural factors. Ignoring this broader context hampers our understanding of health and disease and therefore its treatment.

A couple of years ago, my patients were being seen by a visiting consultant from another hospital while I was on a short vacation. One of my regular patients, a twenty-eight-year-old guy, booked an appointment, complaining of a slight headache. On examination, his

BP was found to be high. The visiting consultant, who was much senior to me, immediately started the patient on BP medication. What would I have done differently in this case?

Well, the patient visited me once I was back from my vacation and told me that the senior doctor had insisted he start taking BP medicine at the age of twenty-eight. That too after a single conversation! Not only did the doctor not ask about psychiatric factors that could very well lead to high BP, he also failed to recommend a significant investigation – for the med buffs, a Renal Doppler (ultrasound). Suffice it to say, the patient is now off the BP meds, exercising well and receiving treatment for anxiety.

Relying solely on reductionist approaches has limited and continues to limit the scope of medical treatments. The possibility of reversing chronic disorders is negated, along with any concept of a cure. What is packaged as 'maintaining your health' really entails daily drugging, allowing pharma companies to make money off of patients for the rest of their years.

Lifestyle modification, holistic therapies and alternative medicine – approaches that consider the whole person – are sidelined in favour of targeted interventions. True to Western medicine *fundas*, the focus is on treating diseases *after* they manifest. This is essential, of course, but it diverts attention from preventive measures. Holistic approaches that account for lifestyle, diet and mental state play a pivotal role in preventing disease, while the reductionist focus has time and again delayed the emphasis on preventive healthcare. This might hinder patients from exploring treatments that could be highly beneficial for their overall well-being.

Thus, while reductionism has undeniably advanced medical science, we need to recognize its limitations. Embracing a more integrative approach that considers the intricate interplay of biological, environmental and social factors is essential for the future of healthcare. Once we acknowledge the pitfalls of reductionism, we can pave the way for more patient-centric and effective medical practices.

In this chapter, you might feel like I am reducing the reduced human further into doshas. Allow me to acquaint you with a few concepts and theories to understand why I continue to stand by doshas and humours.

Humour me, will you?

Cell-centric or Hell-centric?

Western medicine treats the consequence of a disease, not the cause. Reductionist thinking has completely obscured the unity of biological systems. If we were to leave the independent cell in a lab, it will wither and die in no time. But in a Petri dish, it will sustain and multiply. Here is a short summary of the current thought in popular medical culture:

1. The nucleus contains all the genetic material of a cell. It is the supreme commander of the cell.

This concept forms the basis of the central dogma that is taught to us through medical school: the nucleus is the end all and be all of cells. It has long been considered the brain of the cell. Your DNA, which holds your genetic blueprint, lives inside the nucleus. As the DNA helix was unravelled, scientists developed the 'one gene-one disease' hypothesis – the idea that a single genetic mutation is solely responsible for a particular disease. They thought they had finally found the holy grail that would demystify all medical problems to have ever existed. Alas, they were far off.

In 1990, the very ambitious Human Genome Project (HGP) was launched. One of its goals was to decode all known diseases and assign each one to a singular gene. The aim was to decrypt human life down to the letter. However, the researchers found that nearly every single disease had multiple genes governing it – not to mention how lifestyle, food, habits and location governed which genes would be expressed or suppressed. While the one-gene idea was historically important, scientists now see that most diseases result from a complex web of genes, pathways and external factors, rather than a single faulty gene.

Ultimately, this limb of the HGP had to be shut down. Beyond a point, their research was yielding the same information on a loop – that all diseases have multiple genetic components and there is no one gene to blame! There were certain exceptions; genetic diseases which are affected by one single gene like sickle cell anaemia and cystic fibrosis. But these happen to constitute only 2 per cent of all known diseases. That's not to say that the HGP was a failure by any stretch of the imagination. Across thirteen years, it did achieve its goals of gene mapping, gene sequencing and generating open data that provided all genetic information. But the one gene-one disease hypothesis has been largely debunked as most diseases are polygenic (many genes are involved) and multifactorial.

2. The cell is the smallest unit of the living human body. It is the supreme mega-mind that runs the whole body.

Do you want to hear the short version or the long version?

Well, the short version is that no, the cell is not the smallest unit of life.

The longer version requires a deep dive into the flaws of the reductionist approach of Western medicine and how it will continue to be flawed as long as it sees every cell, every organ and every human as a sum of parts rather than a beautifully coordinated, synergistic system. We have come a long way in what we know and understand about cells but the focus is yet to find a mainstream shift.

For a long time, biology taught a simple 'cell theory' – every cell works on its own, the nucleus is the control centre and life is just billions of tiny independent units doing their jobs. But modern research shows that this old idea is far too limited. Cells are not isolated little hermits. Instead, they form a functioning society with one another and their surrounding matrices.

Modern science now concurs that the cell membrane (the covering of your cell) functions as the eyes and ears of a cell – it tells the cell what's going on around it. The nucleus serves as the genetic archive but it does not independently 'control' the cell. A cell doesn't just sit around waiting for the nucleus to tell it what to do. Instead, the cell membrane does a lot of the real-time sensing. It's constantly 'listening' to the outside world, picking up signals like nutrients, stress, temperature and messages from other cells. These signals are then transmitted into the cell and influence gene activation, gene silencing and overall cellular function. So, the nucleus which was so far hailed as the brain of the cell is now correctly estimated to be the gene carrier and not a top-down command centre. Basically the genitals of the cell, not the brain!

Today, we understand the body as a dynamic, networked system where cells, their surroundings and the signals between them all shape how life actually works. This 'surrounding of the cell' is called the extracellular matrix (ECM). If the environment makes the man, then the ECM makes the cell.

The Extracellular Matrix

The ECM is a complex network of proteins and carbohydrates that provides structural and biochemical support to the surrounding cells. It is present within all tissues and organs of the body. In organs, it forms a scaffold that houses cells and helps maintain the structure of the organ. The ECM contains signalling molecules that can influence various cell processes like growth, development and tissue repair. Cells within tissues stick to each other and to the matrix. Otherwise, we would be just a bunch of cells dripping on the floor. Proper cell adhesion is necessary for normal organ function.

The matrix can influence the behaviour of cells, including their multiplication and survival. It gives the cell its functional identity. For instance, muscle cells contract and salivary gland cells produce saliva because their respective ECMs give them that identity and function. When the body is under stress or affected by disease, the functions of cells can change. A cell that is supposed to contract may start storing fat. A cell that is engaged in transportation may pivot to matrix production. (By the end of this chapter I will explain why and how this happens.)

The building blocks of the ECM include proteoglycans, collagen, elastin, fibronectin and laminin. Proteoglycans are giant molecules that give the ECM its gel-like consistency and provide resistance to compressive forces. Collagen is the most abundant protein in the ECM and provides tensile strength to tissues. Another important building block is elastin. Scientists were rather kind to us while naming elastin. It is a protein that gives the tissues – you guessed it – their elasticity and allows them to return to their original shape after stretching. The ECM is the master of modulating organ homeostasis. That may sound fancy, but it basically means getting the organ back to its regular functioning. Say you flooded your liver with booze on Saturday night. The homeostasis mechanisms will give your liver respite and bring it back to normal the next day (hopefully).

Think of the cell as a person. The ECM is analogous to the electricity, maintenance service and telephone connection of their apartment. The capillary (the smallest blood vessel to reach the cells) acts as the water and plumbing system. Together, the cell, its ECM and capillary happen to be the smallest unit of life.

Power Couple: Fibroblast and Macrophage

Fibroblasts are cells in connective tissue that are involved in wound healing and tissue repair. They produce the ECM. On the other hand, macrophages are immune cells that are responsible for engulfing and digesting cellular debris and pathogens. They look after the cell matrix, clearing out dead cells, bacteria and precancerous cells. Fibroblasts are the nurturing, life-giving mothers of the extracellular life of a cell, while macrophages are the protective, hunter-gatherer fathers.

A cell is not disturbed by a disease in isolation. The

surrounding matrix and blood supply are also diseased. In fact, to reach the stage where a disease manifests symptoms requires all the parties involved in maintaining that cell to be affected. Traditional medicine reflects this wisdom, emphasizing the importance of caring for the entire unit of cell and surrounding support tissue – and with it, the human as a whole. Herein lies the beauty of using whole produce, herbs and spices as medication in alternate sciences. Food, unlike pharma drugs, does not fixate on a single cell and cell receptor to work on. Nutrients nourish the ECM, modulate the cell and regulate cell processes. Unlike pharmacological molecules, they do not forcefully subject cells and cell receptors to their whims, suppressing immunity or worse, 'boosting' it.

Just think of it this way: a devotee on his way to Kedarnath or Tirupati walks to his destination on foot – a worthy journey. If he were to be teleported straight to the temple, his soul would not have the chance to be enriched with the bhakti, the shraddha. Undertaking the journey on foot – in the company of millions of fellow devotees, absorbing their energy – while humming praises to the divine, he immerses himself in the spirituality of the pilgrimage. His spirit feels renewed.

This is the nature of the human body, down to a cellular level. The cell is not the centre of the bodily universe just like the Earth is not the centre of the universe. Long before the advent of microscopes, Hippocrates, Sushruta and Charaka saw the body as a connected system. Hippocrates' humoral theory and Charaka's doshas emphasized the importance of internal balance, while Sushruta highlighted the flow of fluids nourishing tissues. Today, we know this 'environment' as the extracellular matrix (ECM). Even without modern tools, these ancient thinkers intuitively understood that health depends as much on the space around cells as the cells themselves.

To this day, the ECM's relationship to health and disease has been undervalued and underrepresented, except by a few scholars of holistic medicine. In my view, the main obstacles are the blinkered view and greed that have shaped Western medicine and pharma corporations. Today's medical training teaches a kidney specialist to see their patient as nothing but a walking pair of kidneys. Not to mention the profit-driven industry of Western medicine, so unlike true holistic medicine.

Another fundamental fallacy of modern medicine is its restricted sample size. The standard reference subject used for research in the West weighs 70 kg, is 180 cm and is a through and through *gora* (of Caucasian descent).[21] Even white women were not included in these studies until quite recently. In fact, it was only in 1993 that the US government mandated the inclusion of women while testing medications that are meant to be universally applied to all adults. One of the reasons given for excluding women was the inconvenience in studying a woman's body because their bodies change constantly through the month due to their menstrual cycle. A reason, in my opinion, that should have driven the scientific community to study the female body even more closely.

Issues with sample size and demographics are just the tip of the iceberg when we talk of flawed clinical studies. Big pharma's approach to getting drugs tested and approved by hook or by crook severely undercuts the production of accurate and universally applicable results. The former editor-in-chief of the reputed *New England Journal of Medicine*, Dr Marcia Angell, has been one of the most vocal critics of clinical studies and their results. In her book, *The Truth About the Drug Companies*, she claimed, 'It is simply no longer possible to believe much of the clinical research that is published, or to rely on the judgment of trusted physicians or authoritative medical guidelines. I take no pleasure in this conclusion, which I reached slowly and reluctantly over my two decades as an editor of *The New England Journal of Medicine.*' She went on to highlight concerns about the marketing, pricing and research practices of pharmaceutical companies.[22] These insights from an actual insider lay bare the deep-rooted corruption – whether conflicts of interest, bias or commercialization – that plagues big pharma.

Anyway, I digress. The key take-away is that we must be cognizant of the limitations of modern science and consider the possibility that the answers to our most morbid health concerns in the twenty-first century have been staring us in the face all this while. We Western medicine practitioners have been brushing aside and outright laughing at Ayurvedic knowledge: doshas, prakruti, vikruti. I had to take a step back and re-examine my own long-standing beliefs to reach the 'heretic' conclusions contained in this book.

Back to the Basics

There are three fundamental, well-founded notions about the human body that we must keep in mind going forward:

1. Each organ in the body is surrounded by its own unique ECM with specific chemical compositions. These matrices play vital roles in regulating organ function and overall health and disruption can lead to disease.
2. Directing drugs specifically to cell receptor sites bypasses the modulatory control by the ECM and interferes with the body's self-regulatory mechanisms.
3. We need to consider the holistic regulation of the organism when designing medical interventions.

Some Hi-fi Science: Nutrigenomics and Nutrigenetics

Nutrigenomics is a branch of science that studies how the foods we eat interact with our genes. It aims to understand how diet can influence gene expression and metabolism; how our food choices influence genetic activity. Food interacts with our bodies right down to the genetic level, leaving an imprint on future generations. The branch of science known as nutritional epigenetics says that what you eat daily can manifest in the form of health or disease even four generations down the line!

Nutrigenetics, on the other hand, focuses on how an individual's genetic makeup can affect their response to specific nutrients and dietary patterns. It looks at how genetic variations can make them more or less susceptible to health conditions like obesity, heart disease, diabetes and certain cancers based on their diet and lifestyle choices. In summary:

Nutrigenomics = How food affects genes
Nutrigenetics = How genes respond to food

Genetic variations can influence how efficiently the body processes and stores nutrients, including fats and carbohydrates. This information can guide weight management strategies – the need of the hour amidst the obesity epidemic. In fact, genetic factors can shape taste preferences, food cravings and satiety. Understanding these factors can help individuals make healthier food choices.

The genetic makeup and eating habits of one's ancestors, even several generations back, can influence an individual's health in myriad ways. Nutrient metabolism – the ability to digest and assimilate certain nutrients – can be inherited too. Dietary habits and food choices within a family – or even a culture – shape those of subsequent generations. This is why I insist on my patients choosing cooking oils that are true to their genetic makeup, rather than what's in vogue in the diet industry.

All that being said, it is time to throw away all that you hold sacred when it comes to genes and their unchangeable nature. While it is true your genetic code is set in stone, how much it expresses itself is completely dependent on your environment. I'd like to turn your attention to the bypass to the genetic code, epigenetics.

Epigenetics

Literally meaning 'above' or 'on top of' genetics, epigenetics deals with modifications that overwrite the genetic information encoded in a person's DNA. These modifications influence how genes are turned on or off without changing the DNA sequence itself. Though these changes can be inherited too, the beauty of epigenetics is that they are reversible.

Epigenetics isn't just fun-to-know info. It plays a crucial role in regulating biological processes, from development to disease. Confused? Not convinced? OK, let me explain this even more simply.

1. **Genes are instructions.** Think of your DNA as a cookbook, in which your genes are a set of instructions. These instructions determine everything about you, from your eye colour to the inner functioning of your body.
2. **Epigenetic marks are Post-its.** Now imagine you're flipping through the cookbook while placing Post-its on certain pages. These notes don't change the actual

recipes (your genes), but they tell you which recipes to pay more attention to and which ones to ignore.

3. **They can turn genes on or off.** Epigenetic marks are chemical signatures that can turn genes on or off. It's like planning your menu for a special meal. Some recipes are used, while others are set aside.
4. **They are influenced by lifestyle.** Your lifestyle – what you eat, how much you exercise, even how you handle stress – can determine where these Post-it notes are placed. Just like you might decide which recipes are more important based on your preferences and the ingredients at hand.
5. **Epigenetics enables adaptability.** It allows your body to adapt to different 'cooking' conditions. For example, if it's hot outside, you might choose recipes that require less cooking (gene expression), like fresh fruits and salads. If it's cold, you might choose recipes that need more heat; soup or comfort food.
6. **You can pass notes to the next generation.** Sometimes, these epigenetic marks can be passed down to your kids. Thus, your cooking preferences might influence how your children approach their own recipes (express their genes).

In essence, epigenetics allows your body to adapt to the environment without changing the actual recipes in your genetic cookbook (DNA).

A real-life example comes from the Bengal Famine of 1943. Millions of people were starved as a result of war-time policies and exploitative economic systems. Pregnant women who experienced severe famine gave birth to smaller children due to the malnourishment. These early-life metabolic adaptations, while life-saving at birth, predisposed them to diabetes, obesity and heart disease later in life. Scientists discovered that while the famine didn't change the children's DNA sequences, it altered how certain genes were expressed. They were 'switched on' or 'off' in ways that affected metabolism.[23] Time and again we have seen such epigenetic marks passed on to the next generation, even influencing grandchildren.

After a bit of hardcore science, let's circle back to ancient medicine.

The Doshas, in Detail

You might notice that the dosha system is vastly different to allopathy's web of super specializations: cardiology for the heart, nephrology for the kidneys, neurology for the brain and so on. This is because it views the body as a whole.

For instance, if a patient presents with bloating, constipation, elevated BP and constant anxiety, an Ayurvedic practitioner would suggest that their vata dosha (transport and communication system) is disrupted. On the other hand, a medico trained in the Western tradition would first target the BP, throw in an antacid and refer the patient to a psychiatrist.

When we address these problems as a group instead of chasing a singular pathology, the role of nutrition emerges beautifully. We cannot dissect our food into independent molecules without taking into consideration where it came from, how it was prepared and the nutrients that coexist within. Nor can we handpick and supplement select nutrients as a blood test deems fit – a very piecemeal approach to nourishing our body. Nutrients work in synchrony. They can complement, supplement or even antagonize one another. These interactions between different nutrients help maintain the delicate ecosystem that is the human body.

While we are on the subject of breaking down food, the more we peer into the microscope, the more we discover different nutrients. Having run out of group names for them we have ended up calling them phytonutrients (nutrients from plants) or antioxidants. Honestly, every plant food has antioxidants – allicin in garlic, rutin in apple peels, resveratrol in grapes, curcumin in turmeric. This overlap has led some people to refer to phytonutrients interchangeably as antioxidants, when they actually serve multiple functions at various checkpoints in the cell's metabolism and growth. But the point remains the same – whole foods are chock-full of nutrition and we don't need a scientist's permission to eat them.

Plants release oxygen not because they love us and want the best for us. They release it because beyond respiration it's their waste product – the oxygen produced in their leaves by photosynthesis will cause injury to the plant cells. That's because oxygen is a through and through extrovert. It wants to mingle with anyone and everyone and is just waiting to accept an electron from any molecule. This reactivity of oxygen is the bane of every living creature as it makes us age and causes inflammation when left unchecked.

While we won't survive an hour without oxygen, its reactivity is the bane of every living creature. The oxygen we breathe sustains life but an errant oxygen molecule causes injury to our cells in the form of free radicals. This oxygen molecule needs to be quelled by antioxidants from our food. When a plant is photosynthesizing, its antioxidant system helps it to keep free radical damage down. When we eat plants, we eat their entire antioxidant machinery that kept its oxygen free radicals in check. These antioxidants keep our free radicals in check, too.

Eat your greens.

The Necessity of Functional Classification

Vata, Pitta and Kapha describe the functional qualities of the human body. Simply put, Vata governs transport and communication, Pitta drives bodily processes towards homeostasis and Kapha forms your tissues and organs. All three are necessary. When any one goes out of balance, the body will do its best to bring everything back to the homeostatic point. Homeostasis is the narrow range in which your body functions best. If an infection raises your temperature by a mere 2 degrees Fahrenheit, you're bedridden. That's how narrow the homeostasis range is.

Here is an analogy to show the practical importance of functionality.

Before zoology was an established science, animals were divided into flying animals (birds and bats), insects, land animals and fish. But as per science, a whale is more closely related to a human than to the shark; a bat is more like a cat than an owl. Mammals - whether they live on land, fly in the air or swim in the ocean - are all one group. Even though this holds true from a scientific perspective, this classification is less than ideal when viewed practically. For instance, if I were to go whale spotting (just imagine I am intending to do that), the fact that the whale is a mammal has very little significance for me. But the knowledge that it is aquatic like a shark is more helpful.

The scientific classification really impressed me in my school days. Mammals in one group, whether they live in the sea or tread the land, birds in one group irrespective of whether they fly or not and - my personal favourite - the cockroach is more related to the shrimp than the salmon. But is all this *gyaan* practically beneficial to a person who is not a zoologist? Not that much.

Similarly, think about how we keep the spices together in our kitchen cabinet based on their utility rather than their scientific classification. These spices could very well have been derived from a seed, a fruit that looks like a seed or a dried root. We store cumin, mustard, saunf and methi daana together for our tadkas even though cumin is from the carrot family, methi from the legume family and mustard from the cabbage family. Not one bit related but always paired together in meals. In everyday life, scientific discrimination isn't that useful or practical.

Allopathic specialties function as taxonomy-like categories: structured and hierarchical, organizing medicine by body systems, disease types and treatment methods. In contrast, the dosha system classifies the body and disorders functionally, focusing on dynamic balance rather than structural divisions.

The Racket of Referrals

The beauty of functional classification is that treatment can begin even before all the science-y mechanisms and nitty-gritties have been figured out. Say a person has a long-standing on and off dry cough. Send him to an ENT specialist and she might detect an irritated sinus. 'Here is your nasal spray,' she'll say. 'Take it twice a day for two weeks and all will be good. Come back if the cough persists and we will take a CT scan of your sinuses.' A lung specialist, on the other hand, is likely to see the signs of allergic bronchitis. 'Indoor pollution,' she might explain. 'A steroid inhaler will do the trick, along with some antihistaminics.' Go to a GP and he could rubbish it all: 'No *baba*, you have acid reflux. One course of antacids and you'll be golden.'

This is the *chakravyuha* of modern medicine - and Abhimanyu cannot escape because he is in the CT machine getting his sinuses scanned!

Am I suggesting that all practitioners of modern medicine are running a big fat racket of referrals, defrauding innocent people and making them broke? No, though there is no denying that there are bad apples in every profession. In the case of these three imaginary specialists I described, the ENT sincerely wanted the patient's cough to go. So did the lung doc and GP. They were conscientious, Hippocratic Oath-abiding doctors who didn't regard him as a walking wallet. They've all had the same foundational education in modern medicine. And yet, their tendency was to see everything through a magnifying glass and amplify their pet organ systems as the one under assault by whatever was causing that cough. The reality is that often, the diagnosis depends on the specialist, not the patient.

If we just leaned closer to listen to the cough and tried to describe it like a five-year-old, we would be closer to the cause. The child would say this:

'Grandma's cough is loud. Like the barking of a dog.' (Sorry, he has a very poor filter. He is a kid after all.)

'Kiddo, does grandma have any gooey spit after she coughs?'

'Nope, it's not an ooey-gooey cough. Just a hoarse barking sound. I can't nap after school because of how loud it is. Sometimes her coughing scares me awake in the night, too.'

So, as per Mr No-filter's account, his grandma is experiencing a dry cough that continues throughout the day. I am a little tempted to agree with the GP ... but does that mean I have to agree with his diagnosis?

We often forget one law of nature: when something bodily is suppressed, whether by disease or deliberately (i.e. through the use of pharmaceuticals), a compensatory mechanism will rev up to return the system to equilibrium. Nature does not agree with disorder. A very popular example you might have seen in movies is a blind person who has developed a keen sense of hearing. The same is true for the inner functioning of the human body. If you are coughing night and day and yet the diagnosis isn't obvious – remember, all three specialists disagreed – it's a good idea to go back to the basics. Let's look at this conundrum as a medical love triangle.

Scenario 1: The ENT's diagnosis is right

Regardless of what incited the cough, it has been irritating the patient's sinus cells. The sinuses drip mucus to lubricate the air passages and protect themselves from the pressure of the cough. That trickle causes the cough to worsen because the throat thinks that the lungs are secreting mucus and the cough reflex is programmed to clear the lungs of any irritant or infection. In the air passages to the bronchial tree, inflammation starts to set in. So, technically, the lung doctor was correct.

Scenario 2: The pulmonologist's diagnosis is right

The lungs have a cough response to the irritant. The pulmonologist takes a detailed history and discovers that the patient was put on antibiotics by another doctor to treat a viral infection. The irritation from the infection left residual inflammation in the lungs – grandma's allergic bronchitis. Fair enough. So, inhaler therapy seems like the right way to go.

Scenario 3: The GP's diagnosis is right

The GP hypothesizes that the viral fever and use of unnecessary antibiotics – since they don't work on viruses – have caused acid reflux. He's bang on about what incited the cough and the post-viral inflammation in the sinuses and lungs, resulting in a dry hacking cough. The GP prescribes a short course of antacids for acid reflux and an antihistaminic to remove the allergy component. The patient recovers within a few days. But wait ... two weeks later, the cough is back.

What just happened?

The antacids suppressed acid production in the stomach and the antihistaminic cleared the air passages from the nose to lungs. However, after the body adapted to this new state of lowered acid production and the patient stopped taking the drugs, she experienced rebound acid hypersecretion and also rebound secretion in the sinuses and lungs. Additionally, antihistaminics that reduce airway secretions impact acid production in the stomach since the receptors are from the same family. Yet another cause for rebound acid hypersecretion.

All three doctors have been proven right; they are not pill peddlers. Yet, their ultra-targeted approach has failed them. Conducting a surgical strike with precise drugs has pushed the patient into a self-sustaining vortex of rebounds. Chakravyuha at its finest. An abundance of accurate information but scant wisdom is at play here.

If we had just listened to the five-year-old's candid recount, we could have kept things simple and identified the symptoms as dry and hot. The patient's diet could have been altered to balance the heat and dryness with cool, moistening foods. The acidity would be tamed gently, the dry inflamed airways moistened. The vicious cycle would break; the rebound mechanisms nipped in the bud. All three specialists are correct – they should be applauded for their excellent diagnostic skills which did not help the patient. But with the holistic approach, grandma's cough wouldn't startle little Mr No-filter awake anymore. Yay, everyone wins!

The diagnostic skills of the three specialists, though excellent, could not help the patient. This wasn't a deliberate racket of referrals, but it reveals some of the foibles of modern medical practice – undermining the sanctity of God-made foods, fixating on an absolute cause of the symptoms and treating it with a singular molecule that may suppress this chief cause but unleash other compensatory mechanisms. This approach often only manages to transfer the baton of disease and diagnosis from one specialty to another.

Where do we stand on this?

At this point, I want to strongly disagree with the idea that modern medicine only treats symptoms. That's simply not true. Modern medicine actually treats the consequences of disease far more than the symptoms. A symptom is what you feel – sneezing, pain, fever, cough. A consequence is what the disease does to the body – inflammation, tissue damage, airway narrowing, high blood pressure, fluid retention, insulin resistance. When a doctor gives you an inhaler for asthma, they're not treating the symptom of breathlessness – they're treating the consequence of swollen, constricted airways. When you take an antihypertensive, it's not to mask dizziness or headaches – it's to reverse the consequences of chronically constricted blood vessels. When antibiotics are used, it's not to ease discomfort – it's to address the consequence of bacterial invasion.

Herein lies the catch. It might sound awesome that Western medicine doesn't chase symptoms as much and goes straight to the pathology. But the journey of the treatment system reaches just that – the pathology, not the pathogenesis (the process by which a disease develops). In fact, it often falls short of the underlying cause of the pathogenesis.

So modern medicine is not merely wiping tears while the fire burns. It is often targeting the fire itself – the physiological changes that make the symptoms appear in the first place. You may feel the symptom improve at first but what is actually being corrected is the biochemical, structural or functional consequence of the disease process. That's far more than symptom control – that's consequence control.

On the other side of the coin, we see irony. Despite being brilliant at tackling consequences, modern allopathic medicine often struggles with true symptom relief in chronic conditions. Patients with migraines, IBS, chronic pain, allergies, autoimmune diseases or long-standing respiratory issues live this reality every day. They're given drug after drug, dose after dose, yet the symptoms pop back up the moment the medicine stops. In many cases, the treatment becomes a lifelong subscription, not a solution.

While this is ongoing, a huge part of modern healthcare culture shifts its focus towards looking good on paper. The goal becomes squeezing every measurable parameter – sugar, pressure, cholesterol, TSH, vitamin levels – into a narrow range defined by a lab report. If your numbers look good, you're told you're fine, even when you feel tired, inflamed, bloated, sleepless, breathless or simply not yourself. It becomes a system obsessed with correcting reports rather than restoring well-being. The disease becomes a set of numbers, and the patient becomes a data point.

This is where traditional systems like Ayurveda take a very different approach. Instead of chasing numbers or suppressing isolated symptoms, Ayurveda looks at the disease progression both upstream and downstream. This means it asks what started the imbalance (upstream) and what it has damaged along the way (downstream). A headache isn't just a headache, it's a clue. Constipation isn't a minor nuisance, it's an upstream blockage. Acid reflux isn't an isolated event, it's a downstream burn caused by deeper digestive imbalance.

In other words, Ayurveda doesn't just plug the hole in a sinking boat. Allopathy can patch the hole brilliantly but the boat is still half-submerged. You're still stuck in the middle of the lake. Ayurveda's approach is different. It takes you out of the lake, drains the boat, repairs the woodwork, strengthens the frame, polishes it and only then does it set you back on the water. It restores the system so the leak has no opportunity to form again.

Traditional medicine is comprehensive by design – that is the biggest takeaway. Even though I have been rooting for traditional medicine to be given a fair fighting chance in our present treatment algorithms, allopathy is what gave me the insight to join the dots. We can by no measure discount the advances in medicine we have made. But if the wisdom of our forefathers is adopted by our present medical systems, we might have a winner!

It is also important to keep in mind that, unlike our three fictional specialists, not all medical professionals are saints who have been blinded by the light of the electron microscope. The modern medical industry was founded on the principles of profit and monopoly. If you are interested in the shady history of modern medicine, look up the Flexner Report (1910). While it was a landmark evaluation of medical education in North America, you should read it with a critical eye. Its recommendations helped standardize and improve the scientific rigor of allopathic medicine but devastated traditional and holistic systems of medicine.

Natural and preventive medicine was pushed to the fringes of healthcare and labelled quackery overnight. Medical licensing laws began to exclude non-allopathic practices. A monoculture of medicine emerged, with little to no emphasis on diet, lifestyle, herbology and holistic diagnosis. One of the biggest donors who enabled this transition was petroleum titan John D. Rockefeller – and not out of benevolence. He saw a way to reshape it around petroleum-derived pharmaceuticals, which his companies could produce in vast quantities. The Flexner Report became the tool that enabled this transformation.

Arthur Sackler, millionaire pharmaceutical marketer and patriarch of one of the most powerful families in the US, has been similarly criticized. In *Empire of Pain*, investigative journalist Patrick Radden Keefe exposed Sackler's complicity in igniting the opioid addiction epidemic in the US in the the 1990s. The book is an excellent starting point to understand the reality of the gatekeepers of modern medicine.

3

THE VATA DOSHA: THE MASTER OF KINESIS

> 'There are, in truth, no specialities in medicine, since to know fully many of the most important diseases a man must be familiar with their manifestations in many organs.'
>
> SIR WILLIAM OSLER

The beauty of Ayurveda is that it does not try to measure the disturbance of a dosha exactly. Depending on the symptoms, the diagnostic route is qualitative. In a world hell-bent on medicating the moment a parameter crosses the 'normal range', this approach is refreshing. Ayurvedic teachings note how a dosha is 'disturbed' or 'aggravated'; that it needs to be 'pacified' or 'modulated'. This is the vocabulary we need to adopt, too. In this chapter and the next, I will elucidate the beauty of this concept and how it aligns with natural healing mechanisms.

In the simplest terms, if there is a roadblock at point A, there will be a guy swearing at junction B because of how bad the traffic is. In a similar vein, when one organ is diseased, another organ system steps up to mitigate the disturbance and bring the body back into balance. A person with a Vata disturbance may have slowed Vata in the gut but heightened Vata in the brain. Think of how anxiety and constipation often go hand in hand. Or heightened Vata both in the gut and brain. Think nervous diarrhoea – something every medico got in the second year of college before their pathology viva.

Vata Dosha – Our Kinetic Bio-energy

Vata is the body's transport and communication system. Our body has a busy network of nerves which innervate every organ and tissue. This is our nervous system and it directs several bodily functions that then fall under Vata.

1. The circulation of blood and lymph, thus enabling the transport of nutrients, oxygen and so on.
2. The production of hormones by the endocrine system that, when secreted, instruct every cell to accomplish a certain fixed function.
3. Hollow organs like the stomach or colon receive orders from the part of the nervous system which isn't under our active conscious mind – the autonomic nervous system. The evacuation of waste products via these organs falls under Vata.
4. It influences speech and sensory perception.

Ayurveda says that the Vata dosha is composed primarily of the air and ether elements. The qualities associated with air include mobility, lightness and dryness, while those of ether include spaciousness and expansiveness. Vata embodies these qualities, reflecting a combination of movement and space.

Individuals with a predominant Vata constitution often have a slender build with light bones and thin, dry skin. They may have prominent joints and a tendency towards coldness in their extremities. Vata types tend to be agile, flexible and quick in their movements. They're known to be antsy and restless by nature. The friend who keeps picking at her skin or rapidly tapping her foot while talking is likely Vata-predominant.

Ayurveda says that Vata is most influenced by the changeable qualities of the autumn and early winter seasons, characterized by dryness, coolness and variability. Vata individuals may experience imbalances during these times, requiring extra care and attention to maintain equilibrium.

I know this might sound like a whole lot of pseudoscience but allow me to elaborate on the timelessness of its application.

Vata at the Organ Level

The brain and sleep

The glymphatic system, a newly identified waste disposal system in the brain, primarily functions while we sleep. Your big, smart brain is so heavy that you would sprain your neck trying to carry it around. To prevent this, God has utilized the buoyancy of the fluid it floats in, cerebrospinal fluid (CSF). CSF is always in circulation within the skull and spine, just like any good plumbing system. The CSF and interstitial fluid (ISF) - fluid between cells - are exchanged to clear out metabolic waste like beta amyloid, a protein linked to Alzheimer's disease. When we sleep, astrocytes - specialized cells in the brain - shrink in size, expanding the space between cells and allowing fluid to flow more freely through the brain's ECM. This mechanism aids in the removal of waste products, supporting overall brain health and functioning.

Parkinson's disease is a neurodegenerative disorder affecting movement, characterized by tremors in the limbs, rigidity and poor balance. It is a hallmark Vata disturbance. The Astrocytes are a type of brain cell which physically shrink night after night to help clear your brain waste. They shrink so the highways are wide open to clear out brain gunk when you sleep. In Parkinson's these cells are no longer able to perform that function. Instead, astrocytes in the region of the brain affected in Parkinson's exhibit compensatory growth in response to pathological changes caused by the disease. This maladaptive response is an attempt by the cells to compensate for neuronal damage and dysfunction. The vicious cycle of malfunctioning astrocytes contributes to the progression of Parkinson's disease.

Mental pursuits and mental health

When I think of a Vata personality, Johnny Depp is the first to come to mind. I'm not referring to his real life but rather his reel life choices; they reflect a certain charming, disarming craziness. A Vata personality can be a creative artist (Willy Wonka), an agile thinker (Captain Jack Sparrow) or a sensitive soul (the Mad Hatter). With a natural inclination towards learning and discovery, Vata types may have a keen interest in intellectual pursuits.

Vata disturbances cause anxiety, racing thoughts and a restless mind. Mental health disorders stem from faulty communication – specifically, problems in the release and uptake of neurotransmitters. Brain cells talk through electrical signals which trigger chemical messengers in the next cell. It's kind of like how ants release tracer molecules in their trail and their fellow ants follow. In Parkinson's, there's a transport glitch; in anxiety, the signals themselves falter.

Gamma-aminobutyric acid (GABA), the brain's natural calming chemical, is often deficient or has poor receptor function in anxiety and epilepsy. The enzyme glutamate decarboxylase (GAD) converts excitatory glutamate molecule into calming GABA, keeping brain activity balanced. When GAD malfunctions, GABA levels drop, tipping the brain towards hyperactivity. This imbalance is seen in anxiety, epilepsy and movement disorders like Parkinson's – all considered classic Vata disorders in Ayurveda.

Digestive system

The quintessential issue during a Vata disturbance is constipation. The muscular movements in the wall of the gut are disturbed, leading to bloating and dissatisfactory emptying of the bowels. As we've discussed, when the functioning of one part of the body is disturbed, it naturally tunes itself in such a way that:

1. It heals the disturbed organ system.
2. The other systems go a little off-calibration to ensure that the disturbed function is taken care of by rest of the body.

Controlling the immune response in the digestive system is crucial for balancing nutrient absorption and protection against bacteria and toxins. Proper digestion requires hyporesponsiveness, i.e. the immune cells in the gut need to stay less reactive to what's within it.

Recently, scientists have discovered that the autonomic nervous system helps regulate inflammation and maintain the gut barrier. While lab tricks can trigger gut stability in various ways, it's sustained by dietary fat in real life. Vata is the body's busy transport system, always on the move. And like a well-oiled machine, Vata is soothed by fats. Oil and ghee calm its restless drive and keep things flowing.

Vata Inside the Cell

The dosha system is not limited to what you see at the level of the individual or organ. Even the organelles within the cells testify to the veracity of this Ayurvedic wisdom.

Microtubules

Microtubules are tiny, cylindrical structures inside cells, made up of protein. They're the support beams that help give cells their shape and structure. They transport important goods around cells, like nutrients, proteins and even genetic material. They also play a role in cell division, helping to pull apart chromosomes when cells need to make copies of themselves. Essentially, think of microtubules as transport and communication highways.

In Alzheimer's disease, there is abnormal accumulation of tau protein – a microtubule-associated protein. This leads to the formation of a dumpyard made of neurofibrillary tangles – abnormal proteins that bulk up the cell. Both tau protein and beta amyloid, which I introduced earlier, are involved in the pathogenesis of Alzheimer's. Tau protein is deposited within nerve cells whereas beta amyloid is deposited around the cells in the surrounding matrix. This disrupts the stability of the microtubule. This destabilization impairs transportation within the cell, further worsening brain degeneration.

Cell membrane fluidity

The cell membrane is a flexible barrier surrounding the cell, made up of fat and proteins. Just like how a balloon can stretch and move, the membrane's shape and flexibility are subject to change. This fluidity is crucial for nutrient and waste movement in and out of the cell. Think of it as a gatekeeper that can adapt to different conditions to keep the cell healthy and functioning properly. Omega-3 fatty acids like ghee and oil (oil is not bad, OK?) modulate the fluidity of your cell membrane. They help strike a balance between a rigid cell membrane that can't function and a wobbly mess that can't hold itself up. The cell needs balance, baby.

For the sake of science and simplicity, I am going to focus on the interaction between one subcellular organelle's functioning and a food to illustrate how Vata shapes health: histone acetylation. But before that, let's drink some vinegar.

Vinegar, the Queen of Condiments

Vinegar has been touted as the best of condiments by Prophet Muhammad, peace and blessings be upon him.[24] It is so versatile and health-giving that humans have been consuming it for centuries despite its distinct sour taste and pungent aroma. While commonly used in the kitchen, vinegar also possesses intriguing metabolic properties that have garnered scientific interest (hi, apple cider vinegar fad). This simple condiment made up of the very beneficial acetic acid and a whole host of good bacteria has a positive impact both within and outside the cell.

When a substance is utilized by the body, it gets converted gradually to different molecules. These are called intermediates. Intermediates, depending on the needs of the body, are either used directly to continue a metabolic process or as raw materials in other metabolic pathways. The key intermediate in the metabolism of acetic acid is acetyl coenzyme A (acetyl CoA). It is a central molecule in cellular energy metabolism and a super-useful molecule that shows up almost everywhere your cells make or use energy.

Acetyl CoA produces energy-carrying molecules such as nicotinamide adenine dinucleotide (NADH) and adenosine triphosphate (ATP). This process provides cells with energy for tasks like muscle contraction and maintains cellular function. The molecules can be converted into fatty acids and cholesterol, which are essential for the cell membrane's structure, energy storage and hormone synthesis.

Vinegar and Histone Acetylation

Histone acetylation is a process your cells use to 'loosen' tightly packed DNA so certain genes can be turned on. Your DNA is closely wrapped around protein spools called histones. The acetylation process helps relax these spools just enough for the cell to read the necessary genetic instructions.

In simple words, histone acetylation is like flipping a switch to turn on genes and make sure our cells function smoothly. It is in fine-tuning this switch that vinegar has a therapeutic effect on metabolic disorders, cancer and neurodegenerative diseases. The production of acetyl CoA from vinegar metabolism contributes to cellular energy production, biosynthesis and gene regulation through histone acetylation. This is nature's finest example of Vata dosha's communication function.

Rasa in Ayurveda and zaika of Unani made life simple. We didn't need to wait for the DNA helix to unfold circa 1953 for humanity to understand the benefits of vinegar. The uncovering of histone acetylation and the brain's glymphatic system in the 1960s and 2000s respectively may have captured Vata's biofunction in action, but the confirmation from modern science came quite late. Rasa in Ayurveda and zaika in Unani had already acknowledged its benefits far earlier and with greater simplicity.

Vinegar is sour and this taste aggravates Vata as per the rasa paradigm. The sour taste increases heat and moisture, which can counterbalance Vata's dryness and coldness. However, the sharp and penetrating qualities of vinegar can also lead to overstimulation and imbalance in Vata if taken in excess.

As a hot condiment, vinegar increases Pitta. It contributes to energy production and heat in the body. Since Pitta controls energy and balance, the sour and heating nature of vinegar can aggravate it, causing acidity, heartburn and inflammation if consumed too much. Drinking vinegar on an empty stomach might boost metabolism, but a little common sense in the morning is better!

Finally, vinegar is beneficial for Kapha dosha. Its sour taste and heating qualities help stimulate digestion and metabolism, which can counteract the heavy, cold and sluggish nature of Kapha. Vinegar can help balance Kapha when used in moderation. I repeat, in moderation.

Based on these insights, Ayurveda recommends the following:

- **Vata**: Use vinegar sparingly and opt for milder varieties such as rice or apple cider vinegar. Don't chug it and/or consume it with just water. Instead, combine it with warming and grounding foods like rice, tuber vegetables and dals in the form of *sirka pyaaz* to get the benefits without disturbing your temperament.
- **Pitta**: Avoid excessive use of vinegar, especially in hot weather or for individuals with strong Pitta characteristics. When using vinegar, opt for less sour varieties and balance it with cooling foods. A refreshing cucumber salad with a vinegar drizzle would be great (more on this later).
- **Kapha**: Vinegar can be included more liberally in the diet to stimulate digestion and balance Kapha's heavy and sluggish qualities. Even so, don't overuse it.

4

THE PITTA DOSHA: THE ENGINE OF THE BODY

Pitta in the Human Body

This dosha eluded me for the longest time. Kapha was the first to untangle in my head and it was a pleasant surprise to see Vata in action at the organ and cellular level. However, Pitta has been my nemesis. Likely because I am a Pitta-type myself, introspection has been hard to come by. It seems fitting that I irritate you a little before this guy comes to the forefront.

The mitochondrion is the powerhouse of the cell. You'll see.

Pitta dosha is considered the driver of all things related to metabolism, energy and maintenance of body temperature. It controls anything and everything that requires energy. The key biomedical players for Pitta are:

- Mitochondria, at the subcellular level
- The endocrine (hormone) system
- The sympathetic nervous system – our body's flight-or-fight guy

- Skeletal muscles – what you call lean muscle mass
- The coating of all your internal organs – the serosa
- Thermogenic fat or the brown adipose tissue
- The source of all energy – the liver and small intestine

The Sympathetic Nervous System (SNS)

This part of the nervous system is responsible for our body's fight-or-fight response. But its work is so much more than that. It is a key player in thermoregulating the body, activating sweat glands and constricting or opening up blood vessels to regulate heat loss. This of course is dependent on the weather. It also plays a big role in metabolism, as it stimulates glucose release, increases fat breakdown and gets your basal metabolic rate (BMR) up during stress or activity. It has a direct influence on hormone release from the adrenal glands (adrenaline and noradrenaline), enhancing energy production. This effect prepares the body for 'fight or flight' – raising the heart rate, increasing oxygen delivery and mobilizing energy stores.

Lean Muscle Mass

Lean muscle mass plays a key role in maintaining body temperature and metabolic health. During physical activity muscles generate heat, making them a major source of thermogenesis. This helps regulate core body temperature, especially in cold conditions. Lean muscle is metabolically active too, supporting efficient energy use and the maintenance of stable blood sugar levels. More muscle mass means a higher resting metabolic rate, bolstering weight management and overall vitality. Building and preserving lean muscle is essential for strength, endurance, metabolic health and thermal regulation.

The Triple Warmer

According to TCM, the serosa and endocrine organs are divided into three zones: upper, middle and lower. The thyroid gland in the upper, the pancreas in the middle and the adrenals in the lower zone. This system is called the triple warmer. I continue to get baffled by the deep insights that have shaped alternative forms of medicine like TCM despite its early practitioners having no access to modern-day knowledge at a microscopic level. Hell-bent on seeing the processes as individual and working in a vacuum with no effect on their neighbours, we have been missing out on what our body as a whole is trying to tell us. The microscope has traded our intuition and observation for shortsightedness. The body's endocrine system and metabolic factory are deeply interconnected, both in the modern biomedical sense and within the Ayurvedic framework. They function together through hormonal signals, cellular energy pathways and thermal balance. The endocrine system regulates metabolism and temperature via hormones. Metabolism is taken care of by hormonal and mitochondrial processes that determine energy usage and heat production. The core conceptual bridge is that Pitta dosha represents metabolic fire (Agni), heat, transformation and digestion – functions that are strongly associated with hormonal and enzymatic activity.

Adrenal glands

Hormones secreted by the adrenal glands like cortisol, adrenaline and noradrenaline activate the SNS, generating heat through fight-or-flight responses. The hormone cortisol supports glucose production and muscle breakdown to produce energy and warmth. Chronically high cortisol causes tissue inflammation, which in Ayurvedic-speak refers to aggravated Pitta dosha.

Ayurvedic correlation: Tejas (the subtle fire aspect of Pitta) is heightened by excess adrenaline. High adrenaline means one's SNS is chronically in overdrive. This state and Pitta-type disorders present in the same ways: acne, gastritis, anger and hair fall.

Pancreas

It releases insulin which regulates glucose metabolism, thus powering mitochondria. Poor insulin sensitivity leads to low cellular energy.

Ayurvedic correlation: Pitta governs digestion and the transformation of food. Metabolic syndrome is a cluster of conditions – like high blood sugar, belly fat, high blood pressure and abnormal cholesterol – that occur together and greatly increase the risk of diabetes and heart disease. The metabolic syndrome which happens to be a disorder with Kapha-Pitta overlap shows Agni imbalance, manifesting as erratic digestion and heat patterns.

Hypothalamus

Sitting in your brain is the ultimate controller of the triple warmer. It works as the thermostat of the body, regulating heat and hunger. It releases hormones which in turn command the rest of the hormone systems. It modulates SNS tone and circadian rhythm.

Ayurvedic correlation: Hypothalamic-pituitary function aligns with the higher control of Agni and Pitta. Disruptions affect the body's hormonal fire, causing irregular periods, mood swings and temperature dysregulation.

Sex hormones

Oestrogen causes vasodilation, which helps in dissipating heat while progesterone increases basal body temperature. You might have heard of checking your body temperature when trying to conceive naturally. Progesterone causes this post-ovulation heating up. The male hormone testosterone directly increases lean muscle mass. This bulking up results in higher metabolism.

Ayurvedic correlation: Pitta governs transformation, including reproductive fire (*shukra dhatu*). We can see that hormonal imbalances manifest in the form of Pitta-type issues: acne, inflammation and period irregularities.

Serosa

Serous layers are thin, double-layered membranes that line internal body cavities and cover the organs within them. These layers include the pericardium (heart), pleura (lungs) and peritoneum (abdomen). They play a critical yet often overlooked role in thermoregulation, immunity and hormonal signalling.

The pericardium cushions and protects the heart from mechanical shocks. It helps in thermal buffering, maintaining a stable environment for cardiac function. It also shields the heart during systemic fevers or inflammation, preventing overheating or excessive inflammation in this vital organ.

The pleura, surrounding the lungs, minimizes friction during respiration and acts as a responsive surface for immune reactions to inhaled pathogens. During infections, it can relay cytokine signals that influence body temperature regulation and breathing rate, critical during fever.

The peritoneum, lining the abdominal cavity, has a rich network of immune cells and is highly sensitive to inflammatory mediators. It plays a key role in metabolic sensing and immune signalling. Infections or inflammation of the peritoneum (for example, peritonitis) can cause systemic responses like fever, altered metabolism and rapid changes in internal body heat. It also participates in hormonal signalling, responding to prostaglandins and cytokines that influence core temperature and digestive functions.

All these serosal membranes are richly supplied with blood vessels and lymphatics, which help transfer heat from internal organs to surrounding tissues and ultimately to the skin, where it can be released. This maintains the body's core temperature during fever, digestion or physical exertion. While not a direct heat-regulating organ like the skin or hypothalamus, the serosa helps stabilize internal heat flow, especially in the internal organs, contributing to the body's finely tuned thermoregulatory system.

Brown Adipose Tissue (BAT)

Often called 'brown fat', BAT is a special type of body fat that helps generate heat without shivering. Unlike regular white fat, which stores energy, brown fat burns calories to keep the body warm, especially in cold conditions. What makes BAT unique is its high concentration of mitochondria – energy-producing organelles – which give it a darker colour and allow it to produce heat efficiently. When you're exposed to cold or experience stress that activates the SNS, BAT gets triggered and starts producing heat to maintain your core body temperature. This process is called non-shivering thermogenesis, meaning your body warms itself up without needing to shiver. BAT is especially important in babies since they need extra protection from the cold, but adults also retain small amounts, especially around the neck and upper back.

Liver and Small Intestine

The liver is named as such because it does everything for you to live. It is like a bustling industrial complex encompassing and managing thousands of factories. Just to scratch the surface, the liver is the seat of heat generation by glucose production and fat oxidation. This guy converts and breaks down hormones and regulates thyroid hormone activation. It also maintains glucose levels and contributes to basal energy expenditure. It is our metabolic powerhouse and hormone buffer.

The small intestine absorbs nutrients that fuel mitochondrial energy production and hormone synthesis. It is the source of the gut-hormone axis and produces hormones like GLP-1, CCK and ghrelin, influencing appetite, energy use and insulin regulation. The gut-associated lymphoid tissue (GALT) contained within it influences inflammatory thermoregulation. The small intestine is the gateway for fuel and hormonal signalling.

As per Ayurveda, the liver and small intestine are the important organs for Pitta. I agree. However, in 1895, German physician Adolf Magnus-Levy also demonstrated the role of the thyroid gland in metabolism. It turns out that the thyroid's function and Pitta's attributes overlap completely.

Connections Between the Thyroid and Pitta

The thyroid gland is the core regulator of the body's metabolic rate and heat. It produces triiodothyronine

(T3) and thyroxine (T4), hormones which increase BMR and stimulate mitochondrial activity, thus contributing to body heat. The hormones that it secretes control growth, development and energy metabolism. Basically, it acts like a 'thermostat' – determining how fast cells work and how much energy the body uses at rest.

If viewed from an Ayurvedic perspective, the thyroid can be strongly linked with Pitta and Agni (digestive/metabolic fire). Excess thyroid hormones manifest in the same way as Pitta aggravation: heat intolerance, sweating, inflammation. Meanwhile, the impact of low thyroid hormones parallels *Agnimandya* (weakening of fire): cold intolerance, sluggish metabolism, *ama* (toxicity).

The thyroid gland produces hormones that regulate the body's metabolism. This aligns with Pitta dosha, which is responsible for digestion and transformation, including metabolic processes. Thyroid hormones help maintain body temperature by influencing the BMR, just as Pitta is associated with heat and metabolic fire (Agni). Proper thyroid functioning ensures adequate energy production and utilization in the body, mirroring how Pitta's fire element contributes to vitality and energy. Though indirectly, thyroid hormones affect digestive health by regulating metabolic rate. Therefore, efficient digestion and nutrient assimilation are key aspects of both thyroid function and Pitta dosha.

Why am I giving the thyroid a special mention? Simply because everyone seems to need a 'boost' in metabolism these days and every other patient of mine has hypothyroidism.

The Inflamed Thyroid

Hashimoto's thyroiditis is the most common cause of low thyroid activity, or hypothyroidism. (Not to be confused with hyperthyroidism, which is thyroid excess.) If you have hypothyroidism, chances are your thyroid gland is burnt out due to relentless inflammation – the hallmark of Hashimoto's. It is an autoimmune disease where the body's immune system mistakenly attacks the thyroid gland. This leads to inflammation and damage, causing the thyroid to produce fewer hormones. Common symptoms include fatigue, weight gain, hair loss, menstrual disturbances, reduced fertility, cold intolerance and depression. Hashimoto's is more common in women and can be diagnosed with blood tests showing high levels of thyroid antibodies and low thyroid hormones. Treatment typically involves daily thyroid hormone replacement medication to restore normal hormone levels and alleviate symptoms.

Daily, I see patients who have been newly diagnosed with hypothyroidism, or those with an old diagnosis coming for a follow up with their thyroid report in tow, wondering if the doctor will increase their dosage of medication or continue it. The allopathic view on hypothyroidism treatment is supplementing the missing hormone with T4, taken on an empty stomach in the morning. Every three to four months, the patient is expected to get their blood tested to make sure the thyroid medication is adequate.

Before Hashimoto's, there was another widespread problem causing hypothyroidism: iodine deficiency-led goitre. Goitre has long been a part of human history. When a patient has goitre, their thyroid gland enlarges to accumulate the scant iodine available in their diet. This is because iodine uptake by the thyroid is a crucial step in hormone production. More than the debilitating medical symptoms, goitre is accompanied by physical symptoms. The big lump in the neck presses on the patient's wind and food pipes, making breathing and swallowing difficult and their voice hoarse. Not to mention the cosmetic disadvantage. You might have seen old pictures of inhabitants from hilly areas with bulbous swellings in the neck. That's goitre and it is caused by iodine deficiency.

Iodine deficiency in the US was a huge problem for the longest time, as many regions did not have any common plant or animal sources of iodine. Close to half the population had swollen necks and distressed thyroid glands. The problem was so rampant that the northern half of the country had earned the nickname 'the goitre belt'. One of the states in this belt was Michigan. In 1924, Michigan was the first state in the US to introduce iodized salt and within a year, it was being sold across the country. After ten years, researchers found that the prevalence of goitre had fallen from 30 per cent to 2 per cent.[25]

The idea of iodination was borrowed from Switzerland, which was the first country to introduce iodized salt. The nation previously had a high prevalence of goitre, since mountainous soils are typically iodine deficient due to deposits being washed away by glaciation and flooding. Such regions also do not have access to seafood, which happens to be a rich source of iodine. We have seen a similar scenario in the Himalayan population. And for that reason, *aapke namak main* iodine *hai*.

Then in the 1950s came another disturbing statistic. The population of the US seemed to be moving towards overdosing on iodine. Wait a minute. Hadn't the US seen a decline in iodine deficiency over ten years, reducing the occurrence of goitre to a paltry 2 per cent? Why hadn't their intervention stabilized there? How did they reach a point of overdose?

Short answer: they increased iodination further. The rationale for this was that higher iodine content would ensure no one was deficient, even if their intake was low. On the other hand, countries like India chose to limit iodine concentration in salt to 20–40 ppm with the intention of protecting the public from iodine excess. Did the US make a big mistake? And was the regular use of supplements and fortifying staples with iodine doing more harm than good?

Well, the direct adverse effects of iodine have been hiding in plain sight. Despite the eradication of goitre and cretinism, there has been a troubling rise in hypothyroidism causing chronic thyroid inflammation.

This translates to a malfunctioning thyroid gland with poor thyroid production – the same outcome seen in goitre. This condition is called Hashimoto's thyroiditis and its cause is still unknown.

The Hypothyroidism Scam

Iodine-iodine everywhere,
All thyroids did shrink.
Iodine-iodine everywhere,
And all on hypothyroidism's brink.

When I was fresh out of my internship, one of the first questions an aunt asked me was, 'Why is my thyroid function low?'

My answer was fumbling, unsure. 'There are many reasons.'

Ask any doctor – regardless of speciality – and their response will boil down to an inadequate and impotent 'It's multifactorial.' If they go into detail about the mechanisms of the inadequate thyroid gland, the medical mumbo jumbo might intimidate or even satisfy you. But again, if you distil it, the answer will lay somewhere along the sad, narrow range between 'People's lifestyles are poor' to 'It's autoimmune.'

Yes, the thyroid is inflamed. In Hashimoto's it is chronically inflamed. But why? How can the scientific community be satisfied with the autoimmune attack on the thyroid being of unknown origin despite such a significant population popping thyroid pills daily for life? Or ... do we already know the answer?

High iodine consumption is the most common cause of hypothyroidism in areas of sufficient iodine. In fact, the rate of lymphocytic infiltration tends to increase in areas where the iodine intake was once low but has since increased due to iodine supplementation. Chances are you, a friend or family member might be suffering from hypothyroidism. If a person has anti-Thyroperoxidase (TPO) antibodies, they have Hashimoto's thyroiditis. TPO is the enzyme that helps take up the mineral form of iodine and make it organic. This process is known as the organification of iodine. When I say autoantibody, I mean an antibody that attacks your own organ – in this case, your thyroid.

In Hashimoto's, there is inflammation because the body is carrying out a relentless, lifelong attack on the thyroid – depleting it, exhausting it. White blood cells swarm and irritate the thyroid, not allowing it to do its job. An anti-TPO antibodies test is often the clincher for a Hashimoto's diagnosis. But this diagnosis is merely a title – we don't have any answers as to the root cause for the presence of this autoantibody. Anti-TPO antibodies are not attacking the thyroid itself – they are preventing the enzyme from allowing iodine to be taken up by the thyroid gland in excess, thus poisoning it. It is indolent inflammation that is destroying the thyroid; collateral damage in the crossfire of antibodies doing their best to reduce iodine organification. And this all may have started because WHO iodinated the life out of your salt.

Salt iodine content should ideally be 15–40 ppm at the household consumption level. If it is regularly much higher than 40 ppm, risk of over-iodization increases. Getting iodine from varied inputs (salt, diet, supplements) may increase risk if overall intake is high – especially for those with known thyroid issues or autoimmune susceptibility. Ironically, patients of Hashimoto's thyroiditis are advised by doctors and online resources to take iodine supplements. The concentration of iodine in some of these supplements is to the tune of over 300 per cent of the recommended daily allowance.

Ideally, salt iodine content should be limited to 15–40 ppm at the household consumption level. Risk of over-iodization increases when it is regularly much higher than 40 ppm. Getting iodine from varied sources (salt, diet, supplements) may increase risk if overall intake is high – especially for those with known thyroid issues or autoimmune susceptibility. Ironically, patients of Hashimoto's are advised by doctors and online resources to take iodine supplements. The concentration of iodine in some of these supplements is to the tune of over 300 per cent of the recommended daily allowance.

The effects of iodine excess have been documented as thyroiditis (thyroid inflammation) and autoantibody formation. Adding more iodine to a hypothyroid patient's diet may be like adding fuel to the fire. Dietary recommendations suggest increasing iodine consumption with rich sources like fish and seaweed, with additional supplements. This is accompanied by a warning to not consume iodine in excess – an excess of 150 mcg to be exact. But the math ain't math-ing here.

- Say you consume 40 ppm iodized salt. You'll need about 5–7 grams of salt per day. But salt consumption trends show that the average Indian or American gets about 9 grams of salt a day.
- Eat marine sources of dietary iodine for an additional 50–200 mcg.
- If you decide to take over-the-counter supplements marketed for thyroid health, you will inadvertently be adding another 150–500 mcg of iodine to the mix.

Take all three sources into account and iodine overdose starts looking far more likely. In fact, some people may be consuming more than 500 mcg per day. Yet the advice of taking iodine supplements and eating marine foods often overwhelms the crucial 150 mcg limit that more patients should be aware of.

In the mid-1900s, the use of iodine-imbued products in other industries – like dairy and commercial baking – began causing a steep incline in iodine consumption in the US. Thankfully, a report from Harvard Medical Publishing in 2011 found that '[t]he situation has stabilized in recent years, with national nutrition surveys showing that most Americans get enough iodine, and only small numbers get too little or too much.'

However, the phenomenon was not simply a localized one. In 1990, a team of Swiss researchers found that '[u]rinary iodine excretion, previously between 18 and 64 micrograms per day, has now risen to 150 micrograms per day.'[26] And this statistic was based on iodine urinary excretion. We have only been taking iodine intake and excretion amounts into consideration. Our physiology isn't as basic as measuring input and output – it does not follow a mathematical model. If we just focus on the starting point and finish line, we miss the entire journey of iodine in the body.

Switzerland intensified both quantity and availability of their iodinated products and led the way for the US to follow. If salt wasn't enough, they added iodine to eggs, bread and milk. All staples have been laced with the poison they have made out of iodine (always remember – the poison lies in the dosage). A mineral which is supposed to be trace is now rather abundant in our diets and bodies. But that begs the question, why is the thyroid gland not in the pink of health as one would expect? And why am I giving you a lesson in government schemes and WHO standards?

It's because something is fishy. Pun intended. And the more you look at it, the stranger it gets. The consequences of chronic dosing of iodine have not been given their due. And why is that? Has there been a deliberate overshadowing of this aspect of thyroid health?

Big pharma has always been rather shady. Let's follow the money, shall we? The global thyroid support supplements market size was estimated at USD 1.87 billion in 2024 and is projected to reach USD 4.08 billion by 2033.[27] In case you aren't aware, the supplement industry is not regulated by the FDA. In fact, they are regulated by no one really. Pharma and supplement companies often pay for the studies that test their own products, which means the research can sometimes be designed or interpreted in ways that make the product look better. This creates a conflict of interest, since the people funding the research also stand to profit from the results. There are definitely gaping holes in hypothyroid dietary recommendations and more questions than ever. Why hasn't there been a more rigorous follow-up of iodine levels in those with Hashimoto's? Have big pharma and regulatory bodies contributed to the lack of solid dietary guidelines?

By now you must have guessed my speculations in the light of industry lobbying. Everyone scratches each other's backs. One widely known example of the government looking the other way in matters of public health has been lead. The US government has been complicit in poisoning its own people and by virtue of being the masters of the world, everyone else too. Reports of chronic lead poisoning and brain dysfunction from canned foods and leaded paint were first made public in the mid-1800s. But the US government didn't get lead out of paint and petrol until 1978. A lag of close to a century!

The US government has done a great job in eliminating goitre. But was that enough for thyroid health? It baffles me that iodine is placed on a pedestal and treated as the end all and be all of thyroid health even though evidence toes the line of even mild overdoses causing thyroid inflammation over time.

At this point, I have to acknowledge the difficult situation that all doctors have been faced with. The peddlers of illness who shaped our syllabus never taught us to advise the patient to check their intake of iodized salt. And even if a patient resorts to reducing iodized salt intake on reading this book, where will they find iodine-free salt? Pink salt? I wouldn't recommend that for regular consumption either. I have seen patients present with high potassium after making this sudden swap and the consequences are way worse than high sodium. This situation is a gift that keeps giving to big pharma, keeping us sick and trapped in the system.

TSH on a High Throne

Thyroid-Stimulating Hormone (TSH) is produced in the brain. It instructs the thyroid to produce and release hormones into the bloodstream. When thyroid hormone levels are low, the pituitary gland releases more TSH to boost hormone production. Conversely, if thyroid hormone levels are high, TSH production decreases. Essentially, TSH levels work as a surrogate for thyroid function. I repeat, as a surrogate. A pretty good one, at tracking thyroid function, but a surrogate nonetheless.

In modern medicine, TSH has been treated as the ultimate controller of the thyroid gland. Even though TSH does regulate thyroid hormone production, this is an oversimplification of how the thyroid works. The thyroid's hormone-producing unit is a follicle, filled with a substance called thyroglobulin. These follicular cells sit in a tight, circular huddle around the pool of thyroglobulin, each one facing inward like attentive guardians keeping watch over their shared nursery. When the body signals a need for thyroid hormones, these follicular cells reabsorb the thyroglobulin from that pool, attach iodine to it and enzymatically sculpt it into active T3 and T4. The finished hormones are then released into the bloodstream. It's a delicate, almost maternal process – thyroglobulin giving a part of itself to nourish the rest of the body.

But just like any stay-at-home mother, thyroglobulin has been ignored and disrespected by science. This chunky protein which is always, always, always in surplus in that huddle hasn't been given its due. The thyroid hormone is the caretaker of each and every cell of your body and supervises pretty much every cellular function. Thyroglobulin, always available in plenty within the follicle, stays ready to ramp up hormone supply as required. In a normal thyroid, thyroglobulin is released into the bloodstream in small amounts due to physiological leakage from follicles and ongoing hormone synthesis. However, when the thyroid is chronically inflamed – as seen in hyper- or hypothyroidism – two things happen. First, thyroglobulin is exposed to the bloodstream in a more significant way. Second, the inflammatory cells relay the ongoings of the disturbed gland to the immune system. This increases the severity of the attack on the follicles, giving rise to anti-thyroglobulin antibodies.

There are a lot of ignored facts about this stay-at-home protein's function, apart from simply being the thyroid hormone's mum. It constantly looks after the well-being of the thyroid, telling cell huddles when to take rest or get active. It stops its own production if the thyroid hormone is sufficient and spikes it when there is a greater demand, as seen during puberty and pregnancy. Sitting on its high throne, TSH isn't even aware of the activities of thyroglobulin because it is only affected indirectly by circulating hormone molecules (remember, it's a surrogate marker for thyroid status). The huddle has a basal layer which is in contact with the external blood and affected by TSH but thyroglobulin sits at its apex, managing the workings of the thyroid from the inside.

Despite its crucial role, there is hardly any literature with more than a scant mention of thyroglobulin as the functioning CEO of the thyroid. It works locally via a short loop feedback mechanism while TSH, the alleged CEO of the thyroid, is given all credit.

We have been drawing kindergarten-level loops from the thyroid to the pituitary gland to explain the feedback mechanism of hypothyroidism to our ailing patients: the more the TSH, the less the thyroid hormone in your body and vice versa. It is not as simple as that. Hormones are intricately linked to the time of day, the foods you've been eating, the exercises you've been doing, the fights you've been fighting, the stresses you are under, the menses you've been bleeding and the age you've been hiding. For a more nuanced interpretation of these mechanisms, we can go back to the functional bio-energies or doshas. Yes, I am going to take help from 'complementary medicine' to simplify thyroid health for you.

Pitta Inside the Cell

The mitochondrion is the cell's central unit of hormonal action and heat production. The thyroid hormone, cortisol and insulin act on mitochondria to regulate energy output and heat. Dysfunction leads to reduced heat production, fatigue and inflammation. From an Ayurvedic perspective, the mitochondria is the centre of cellular Agni. Weak mitochondrial function translates to depletion of Pitta, showing up as cold hands and feet and indigestion. Overdrive, on the other hand, causes high Pitta and with it, inflamed skin, heat intolerance and hyperacidity.

Pitta Dosha in Action

I want to reiterate that the dosha system is a functional classification. So, if you have a pitta aggravated state you might have acne and red skin, along with a helping of acidity. In this section I will detail pitta disturbances by symptom rather than cause. Drawing parallels with biomedicine, I will suggest foods that can naturally give relief.

Inflammatory acne

Before reaching for retinoic acid and antibiotic creams, we need to fix ongoing bodily disturbances to tackle acne. All the Pitta dosha organ systems are involved in causing the eruption on your face. Regardless of whether the chicken came first or the egg, the end result is acne. Therefore, our focus should be cleaning up our systems – from inciting cause to disturbed function to obvious effect. Capiche?

1. The **sympathetic nervous system** alters sebaceous (oil) gland activity via adrenergic signalling. It also modulates blood flow and immune activity in the skin. Chronic SNS activation due to stress, poor sleep and stimulants (like excess caffeine) leads to increased oil production and inflammation. This causes delayed healing of the skin barrier. The skin pH is also altered, instigating an increase in acne-causing bacteria – *Propionibacterium acnes.*

   Food Modulators:
   - Ashwagandha – blunts cortisol spike
   - Tulsi – reduces adrenal hyperactivity
   - Pumpkin seeds – magnesium-rich, calms nervous system

2. **Mitochondria** are involved in programming the death and regeneration of skin cells – sebocytes and keratinocytes. Mitochondrial dysfunction increases lipid peroxidation of sebum and triggers an immune

response that causes inflamed pustules on the skin.
Food Modulators:

- Amla (Indian gooseberry) – rich in vitamin C and polyphenols that support mitochondrial function
- Moringa leaves – anti-inflammatory, high in quercetin and chlorophyll
- Fermented foods (e.g., kanji, rice gruel, buttermilk) – support mitochondrial health via the gut-brain-skin axis

3. Both under- and over-functioning of the **thyroid gland** can cause skin flare-ups. Hypothyroidism leads to reduced skin turnover, which means cells are not systematically dying and regenerating to maintain a balance. This leads to dull, thickened skin and the formation of comedones. In hyperthyroidism we see overactive sebum production causing oily skin and acne.
Food Modulators:
    - Coconut oil – boosts thyroid T3 activity and reduces inflammation
    - Iodine from natural sources such as seaweed in moderation
    - Sesame seeds – zinc, selenium and tyrosine-rich, aiding hormone balance

4. **Lean muscle mass** has a surprising role to play in acne. Inactivity increases insulin and androgens which leads to sebum excess. Poor muscle tone causes systemic

inflammation and low detoxification. Exercise supports lymphatic drainage and muscle tone.

Food Modulators:

- High-quality plant proteins (e.g., moong or urad dal) – support muscle and insulin sensitivity
- Fenugreek seeds – improve glucose metabolism
- Millets – balance blood sugar and support lean muscle mass

5. **Serosa** – the lining of the internal organs – prevents leaky gut and inflammation that can trigger skin eruptions. A leaky gut can lead to endotoxemia – translocation of bacterial products into the blood. This leads to skin inflammation. The processed food lobby has been pushing hard to make us believe that chocolate, pizza and fries don't cause skin breakouts. Since the 1990s, much effort has been put to shift the blame from internal imbalance only to skin bacteria. This means you binge on ultra-processed foods, get angry acne and then reach out for a seven-step skincare routine to undo the damage – a foolproof money-making machine that benefits more than one industry. The fact remains that excess dietary fat or refined carbs irritate the gut lining and increase systemic inflammation. Chronic low-grade inflammation in serosal linings burdens the detox pathways of the liver and skin.

   Food Modulators:

   - Buttermilk (chaas) – probiotic, anti-inflammatory, strengthens gut lining

- Tender coconut water – cools serosal heat, hydrates gut mucosa
- Coriander seed infusion – anti-inflammatory for the gut, clears heat

Gastritis

In conditions like gastritis and acid reflux, several systems contribute to symptom development. The serosa, particularly the gastric mucosa, becomes inflamed due to internal heat, spicy foods and irritants. The SNS exacerbates the issue by increasing acid production under stress. Mitochondrial dysfunction caused by oxidative stress in the stomach lining impairs cellular repair and energy balance. Additionally, overactive thyroid function may heighten metabolic activity, leading to greater acid output and further aggravating the condition.

Migraines

Migraines accompanied by light sensitivity are often linked to multiple underlying dysfunctions. The SNS can trigger vascular instability, contributing to the throbbing pain experienced. At the cellular level, reduced mitochondrial energy metabolism in neurons decreases the brain's ability to manage stress and stimuli. In Ayurveda, Pitta dosha imbalance causes heat to rise towards the head, worsening symptoms when exposed to light or hunger. The serosa, particularly via the gut-brain axis, may also play a role in triggering attacks.

Heat intolerance

Heat intolerance and excessive sweating are common signs of an overactive thyroid gland, which accelerates metabolism. The SNS enhances thermoregulatory responses, further increasing sweating. Mitochondria in such cases become hyperactive, generating excess body heat. The serosa, particularly in the gut, may respond to this internal heat with increased permeability, potentially leading to systemic inflammation or digestive discomfort.

Foods that can help tackle these symptoms

Here are some foods that can help modulate the SNS, thyroid, mitochondria, skeletal muscle and serosa to reduce acne holistically:

1. Amla juice and guduchi powder – strong antioxidant support for mitochondria and skin; support thyroid metabolism and reduce heat
2. Buttermilk, roasted cumin and mint – cool the SNS and serosa, support the gut, mild detoxifiers, balance Pitta
3. Soaked fenugreek, coconut and curry leaves chutney – regulate glucose, improve thyroid and liver metabolism, reduce oxidative stress, support muscle tone
4. Moringa and moong dal khichdi – balance Vata-Pitta, rich in sulphur compounds (good for skin), improved detoxing and muscle recovery

5. Tender coconut water and coriander seed water (taken in the morning) – cool serosa and reduce gut inflammation, support electrolyte balance, modulate thyroid output gently

5

THE KAPHA DOSHA: THE AGENT OF ANABOLISM

The true essence of man is matter. In Hindi, Urdu, Kannada and many other Indian languages, the word 'kapha' means phlegm. It is true that when the Kapha dosha is imbalanced, there is mucus overproduction and congestion in the respiratory tract. But that happens to be a gross oversimplification of this dosha's impact on health. Let's think of this dosha in a functional rather than taxonomic manner.

Kapha dosha is the mason who builds your body. If Vata is the contractor, Kapha is the handyman. The scaffolding that holds the cells in our organs is laid down and maintained by the Kapha dosha. It keeps the skin and mucous membranes moisturized. Children have a predominance of Kapha dosha irrespective of their prakruti (nature) because their bodies are growing and developing and their food needs to be diverted into growth and anabolism (tissue building). It is for this reason that children are more susceptible to mucus congestion in the chest than adults.

In Ayurveda, Kapha is said to be of the earth and water elements. It governs structure, stability, lubrication and immunity in the body and mind. Heavy, cool, slow, oily and dense – these key characteristics make Kapha responsible for physical strength, tissue formation and emotional calm. When balanced, Kapha promotes strength, stability and a sense of calm.

Kapha is the umbrella term for anabolism. Anabolic functions are the body's building processes – they help you grow new tissues, repair muscles, make hormones and store energy for later use. Think of it as your body's 'construction mode', where it takes nutrients and turns them into stronger muscles, bones and cells. It provides structure to the body by contributing to bones, muscles, tendons and other tissues. Kapha ensures that joints are sufficiently lubricated, preventing stiffness. This is important especially for arthritic patients whose joint function worsens in winters. It is also involved in cell growth, repair and regeneration.

When Kapha is imbalanced, a person might experience congestion, lethargy, water retention and depression. This disturbance often results from overeating, lack of exercise, cold weather or excessive sleep. Stimulating activities and the consumption of warm and light foods – while reducing heavy, oily or cold substances in the diet – can help manage Kapha. Keeping this dosha in balance supports vitality, emotional clarity and a healthy immune system.

In Unani, the concept of Kapha corresponds to the

humour called balgham (phlegm). Though there is no direct concept of Kapha in TCM per se, its qualities closely align with a combination of the spleen and lung systems, as well as the concepts of dampness and phlegm. Putting together Ayurvedic, Unani and TCM concepts, Kapha equals balgham equals spleen and lung dysfunction equals dampness and phlegm accumulation. Treatment principles in all three medical systems emphasize warming, drying and stimulating strategies to reduce excess and restore balance.

Kapha in the Cell

The Kapha dosha manifests at the subcellular level as the rough endoplasmic reticulum (RER), golgi apparatus and secretory vesicles. These are the main organelles involved in producing the extracellular matrix. The RER synthesizes ECM proteins such as collagen, elastin and proteoglycans. The golgi apparatus modifies and packages ECM proteins and glycoproteins. It also adds carbohydrate chains to proteoglycans and glycoproteins, important for ECM structure. The secretory vesicles transport processed ECM components from the golgi to the cell surface, where they are secreted into the extracellular space. These organelles work together within cells – primarily fibroblasts, chondrocytes and other connective tissue cells – to produce and secrete the complex mixture of proteins and carbohydrates that form the ECM. This is how the structure of the internal organs is maintained by Kapha.

Kapha at the Organ Level

Spleen

The spleen plays a vital role in maintaining blood integrity by filtering out aged or damaged blood cells, ensuring that only healthy, pliable cells are circulated. It also functions as a platelet reservoir, releasing them into the bloodstream when needed – for instance, during injury – to support clotting and prevent bleeding.

It also happens to be a key immunological organ. The spleen houses immune cells like macrophages and lymphocytes that help regulate inflammation and protect the endothelium from damage, especially during immune stress or infection. Although it doesn't directly control electrolyte balance like the kidneys, the spleen indirectly supports fluid stability by recycling haemoglobin and plasma proteins. This process contributes to maintaining colloid osmotic pressure within blood vessels, preventing fluid leakage and edema (fluid retention).

Kapha parallels the spleen's role in fluid metabolism and nutrient transport in TCM. When the spleen is weak, it fails to transform and transport fluids properly, leading to damp accumulation – a concept that is very similar to Kapha excess.

Leaky gut is increasingly common today because stress, processed foods, antibiotic abuse and poor sleep patterns weaken the gut lining. When this barrier becomes 'leaky', bacterial fragments and toxins enter the bloodstream – similar to how Ayurveda describes ama, the toxic byproducts of weak digestion. These circulating toxins force the spleen to work overtime as the body's immune filter. Meanwhile, fatty liver – a very common finding thanks to processed foods – slows down hepatic and splenic blood flow. Together, this constant immune load and sluggish circulation create low-grade inflammation, insulin resistance and hormonal imbalance. Over time, these changes converge into what we now call metabolic syndrome.

Lungs

According to TCM, the lungs play a key role in regulating water passages, managing fluids and governing *Qi* (pronounced chee) – a central concept that loosely translates to 'life force', in the same vein as Ayurveda's *Prana*. When the lungs' Qi is weak, phlegm and dampness accumulate in the respiratory system, akin to Kapha-related issues like congestion, heaviness and slow metabolism.

This view holds up when we turn to modern science. Lungs aren't just useful for breathing. Healthy lung mechanics and deep diaphragmatic breathing are super important for efficient lymphatic drainage. Lymphatics are a network of vessels in the body that help remove waste, toxins and extra fluid while also supporting the immune system by transporting infection-fighting cells. When lung function takes a hit during respiratory illnesses, symptoms include poor lymph flow, congestion all over the body, edema and inflammation. Kapha dosha is, in essence, keeping the hardware of the body in working condition. This includes the cell, surrounding matrix and circulatory system – both blood and lymph vessels. Disease takes hold in human tissue only when all of these have been disrupted.

Bronchitis, due to viral infection or allergies, leads to chest congestion that affects the airways and digestive system locally. The airways become inflamed and filled with thick mucus, narrowing air passages. This makes deep breathing difficult, causing people to instinctively take short, shallow breaths. Addressing inflammation, clearing mucus and practicing breathing exercises (like diaphragmatic breathing) can help restore lung function. Impaired lung mechanics can reduce chest wall movement and the negative chest pressure causes lymph and venous blood to move upward towards the heart. This mildly impairs lymphatic drainage, especially in sedentary patients or during acute flare-ups, contributing to fluid retention. In chronic lung diseases, this mechanism is overwhelmed and the fluid retention in the body is more pronounced.

Traditional home remedies can mitigate the vicious cycle of hyperresponsive airway in a gentle manner. One can use warm, healing herbal decoctions. For example, tulsi to clear the respiratory tract, mulethi to soothe inflamed mucosa and ginger to improve circulation and dissolve mucus.

Steam inhalation with eucalyptus or ajwain vapours can help loosen chest congestion, open nasal passages and reduce heaviness in the head. Gentle expectorants like a small amount of honey mixed with black pepper thin out phlegm so that it is easier to expel.

Finally, support lung-prana movement through chest-opening practices such as pranayama (deep, rhythmic breathing to expand the lungs) and nasya (oiling the nasal passages), keeping the upper respiratory channels moist, clear and protected.

Kapha and Metabolic Disorders

All metabolic disorders fall under the umbrella of Kapha dosha disturbance. If you adjust the lens and take a closer look, these disorders have the same first hit: the abnormal deposition of raw materials in organs.

Fatty liver

When a person eats more than their body utilizes over a long period of time, they are bound to develop insulin resistance. This directs the liver to accumulate fat. Fun fact: fat is supposed to be stored *only* in adipose tissue (fat cells) and nowhere else. If it is collecting in your liver or pancreas, you need to move more and eat less.

Such rogue fat accumulation causes a lot of changes at the molecular and cellular level. After the first hit of insulin resistance, there is a stark shift in the function of one type of liver cell, the hepatic stellate cell. It changes its function from vitamin A production and storage to producing the ECM.

If you feed your body enough fuel, it will go into hoarding mode. Note how I say fuel and not food. When food is in excess, it starts to behave more like a toxin than a source of nourishment. Not to mention that the processed junk we put in our bodies scarcely resembles real food. When the liver cells are disrupted by excess food, their natural function changes to an adaptive one at best – tucking away excess fuel to deal with the barrage of food. The stellate cells, having changed their modus operandi to take care of the fuel excess, end up laying down more and more ECM and converting empty carbohydrates into triglycerides. These triglycerides (tri – three, glyceride – glucose molecules) make up the 'fat' affecting the fatty liver.

The second trigger that causes the liver to become fatty is oxidative stress. A typical patient of fatty liver may look nourished or overnourished but they are actually nutritionally deficient. Without a good diet, the body gets sparse nutritional support. The problem continues to worsen due to a lack of antioxidants from fresh fruits and vegetables – highly necessary to clear the metabolic mess that excess eating caused in our organs. The ongoing inflammation starts to remove the damaged liver cells. These changes collectively cause a vicious cycle which ends up recruiting more liver cells into handling the fuel overload or die trying.

Both Ayurveda and allopathy agree that the liver's function declines because of fatty liver. However, Ayurveda attributes fatty liver to a Kapha disturbance.

The abnormal ECM production due to stellate cell dysfunction equates to an increase in Kapha. The same things that balance the Kapha dosha also balance the fatty liver – mindful eating and increased physical activity. With timely intervention, you can even reverse the fatty liver progression and bring the organ back to normal.

Thyroid and insulin resistance

At the intersection of the metabolic controller–thyroid and metabolic resistance–diabetes, Pitta and Kapha cross paths. Let me briefly summarize the link between diabetes and hypothyroidism.

1. Insulin resistance can develop due to excess protein intake – something we're seeing across the world today.
2. Insulin resistance affects thyroid function by altering activity of the deiodinase enzyme, which converts the less active thyroid hormone (T4) to the more active form (T3). Insulin resistance also reduces thyroid hormone uptake in tissues.
3. Excess thyroid hormone increases blood glucose levels, starting the cascade that leads to insulin resistance. Even the inflamed thyroid gland of Hashimoto's starts off with hyperthyroidism, as the injured thyroid gland ends up leaking its hormones.
4. Hypothyroidism causes insulin resistance thanks to altered glucose and fat metabolism, inflammation and impaired insulin receptor function. In simple words,

both hyper- and hypothyroidism lead to diabetes.

5. Biochemical studies have shown that insulin stimulates albumin production in the liver. Excess protein causes an increase in prealbumin, albumin and globulin – the protein molecules in our blood which the thyroid hormone attaches to. An increase in these proteins means the thyroid hormone is more tightly bound, making it less available to the tissues for use. Also, TSH becomes spuriously high because it cannot detect much free thyroid hormone. The surrogate marker ain't all that accurate when it comes to thyroid health.

You know what ... perhaps I cannot be brief with this topic, especially after being critical of protein intake in points one and five. I hope you can excuse me for cancelling protein once you hear my case.

Excessive consumption of proteins, particularly those that abound in branched chain amino acids (BCAAs), leads first to insulin resistance and then diabetes. What foods have plenty of BCAAs? Ahem, meat, milk products, eggs, soy and legumes. All your richest sources of protein are full of BCAAs. Are these amino acids bad? Absolutely and emphatically NO! But you already know what I'm about to say, right? The poison lies in the dose. Your protein powder is making you diabetic.

Gosh, I've really opened Pandora's box by condemning protein, haven't I?

The Protein Lobby

There was a flurry of research from 2019 onwards into the association between high protein intake and insulin resistance.[28] Most of these papers came to a very impotent conclusion – that there is a weak association between high protein intake and insulin resistance.

The truth is that when we keep guzzling protein in the form of shakes, egg whites and tofu this and that, it puts a strain on the insulin in our system. Insulin plays a central role in the way the body handles food and protein is no exception. It stops protein from breaking down, helps your body build and keep muscle, and recover after exercise or injury. Too much protein makes insulin work overtime and eventually leads to insulin resistance – just the way excess carbs do.

There should be a bright red notification flashing 'Too much protein can worsen diabetes', but I haven't seen one yet. Most guidelines only emphasize that higher protein intake offers no added benefit for muscle growth or metabolism once you reach an adequate amount. Warnings against high protein intake are largely limited to kidney patients. Why do influential scientific bodies remain non-committal instead of publishing a strict guideline for this? Two words: protein lobby.

The influence of the protein industry on dietary guidelines is fraught with lobbying, conflicts of interest and industry partnerships. While organizations like the FDA, Centers for Disease Control and Prevention

(CDC) and ADA claim to provide evidence-based guidance, the involvement of industry stakeholders has a very direct impact on the development of their diet recommendations.

For instance, during the development of the 2015 Dietary Guidelines for Americans, food and beverage (F&B) companies and trade associations lobbied the US Congress aggressively, spending over $77 million on lobbying activities.[29,30] These efforts included advocating for policies that would benefit their products by promoting higher protein intake from animal sources. A paper published in 2022 found that industry lobbying has thoroughly compromised WHO's global health governance system. Producers of goods like commercial milk formula and processed foods have ramped up efforts to influence WHO policies.[31]

A Balancing Act

At this juncture I would like to introduce a concept which is so flagrantly ignored in modern medicine: hormesis.

Hormesis is a biological phenomenon wherein a substance exhibits different effects depending on its concentration. At very low levels, the substance may have little or no effect; at low-to-moderate levels, it can trigger beneficial adaptive responses; and at high doses, it becomes inhibitory or toxic. This creates a biphasic dose-response curve with a narrow 'beneficial window', where modest exposure is stimulatory but excessive exposure is harmful.

Let me simplify this with a few common examples.

1. If the pH of a substance is very high (alkaline) or very low (acidic) it behaves in the same way – extremely corrosive.
2. You've just completed Thyroid 101, so you might realize that hormesis is glaringly obvious in the case of iodine. Deficient iodine and you get hypothyroidism and a goitre hanging from your neck. Increase the iodine as a result of government implemented schemes and you might get a flatter inflamed gland and yet again, hypothyroidism.
3. Getting the hang of it? Cool! Low protein causes muscle wasting and negative nitrogen balance (i.e., you excrete more protein than you consume). Eat protein in excess long enough and insulin resistance will not let you retain it.
4. Low carbs cause decreased cognition and brain function. High carbs cause insulin resistance, which also affects your mental health and cognition.
5. Hypoglycaemia (very low blood glucose) and hyperglycaemia (very high blood glucose) both present in the same ways: loss of consciousness, extreme weakness and possibly a coma, depending on severity.

Hormesis challenges medical models that assume a linear dose-response relationship, where the impact of a substance is constant regardless of dose. It challenges the claims of the entire supplement industry. There is a dire need for a more nuanced approach to evaluating the safety and efficacy of these pills. Drugs are assigned an accepted dose, above which they are toxic and below which they are inadequate. But nutrient supplementation has not been treated the same. Our bodies require trace minerals in traces, not in abundance.

Hormesis also has a place in the ageing process and longevity. Mild stressors, such as caloric restriction, fasting, exercise and low-dose exposure to toxins (yes, you read that right), promote longevity by activating protective and repair mechanisms. Even the cold plunges that have become so popular via social media and podcasts are rooted in hormesis.

If you have a finance or maths background, you can understand hormesis as being a bell-shaped curve. The highest point represents the best result and in the end, everything balances out. This curve shows that there's an optimal amount for everything. Too little means you're deficient, moderate is the sweet spot and too much becomes harmful. Simply put, moderation is key. Or, as I say it, average is awesome.

The supplement and pharma industries, protein powder-peddling podcasters and so-called food 'experts' armed with polarizing diets to make your problems go away have one thing in common. Their products and advice all follow the same approach – the more the better! In reality, nature isn't linear. It is a bell-shaped curve. But you can't make a trillion-dollar industry or rake in millions of views by recommending moderation.

Sannipata: The Three Doshas Meet

Interstitial lung disease (ILD) is a group of respiratory disorders that affect the lung's support tissue. This interstitium surrounds the alveoli – tiny air sacs in the lungs. When it gets injured due to internal or external factors, an abnormal healing process is triggered. This leads to scarring and thickening of the interstitial tissue, making it harder for oxygen to enter the blood. Environmental pollutants, autoimmune diseases or infections contribute to the development of ILD.

In an effort to reverse the harm done, the body fights back and the lungs end up becoming chronically inflamed. With inflammation constantly adding fuel to the fire, the wound healing response also cascades. It's a slippery slope of sorts; the inflammation that was supposed to put out the fire now commits arson itself. Despite the efforts of the immune system, the lungs cannot be restored to full health. What the body ends up with instead is inflammatory cells infiltrating the lung tissue, leading to the production of fibrotic scar tissue. Over time, the unrelenting damage and consequent scarring keeps reducing the functional area within the lungs. This progression eventually leads to respiratory failure.

The pathogenesis of ILD involves chronic inflammation and abnormal wound healing processes within the interstitium of the lungs. If you have caught the drift of the doshas, you can easily deduce that this is a Kapha disorder. The entire progression mirrors the Kapha disturbance we saw in the fatty liver, with the excess fibrotic tissue acting as a starting point. However, as per Ayurveda, the other doshas are also affected by ILD. Pitta happens to be disturbed because of the untiring inflammation. Vata is affected because the oxygen transport by the lungs takes a hit.

Here comes the brilliance of the functional classification of diseases.

Although the triggers of ILD have increased Kapha and Pitta, the disease ultimately manifests as a loss of air exchange surface area. The sac-like lung alveoli get progressively destroyed by abnormal interstitium production. The result is less oxygen transfer from the lungs to blood. In effect, the Vata function – transport of oxygen – is impeded.

This disease process is beautifully described in Ayurveda as a Sannipata disorder with Vata dosha in a Kapha seat. Sannipata means all three doshas are affected at the onset of disease. As the disorder worsens and symptoms start to appear, we see all the tissue functions – anabolism (Kapha), metabolism (Pitta) and system dynamics (Vata) – getting disrupted. Vata dosha in a Kapha seat means that even though the root of the problem is a Kapha disturbance, the affected function is Vata.

Vata dosha is a normal force of movement in the body, present in everyone. It is the kinetic energy giving a dynamic outcome. When a person is healthy, it functions smoothly. However, when Vata is grossly disturbed as in ILD, this natural state is amplified, leading to emaciation, anxiety, acid reflux and chronic indigestion. When Vata flows, life moves; when it rages, the body withers.

Modern medicine prescribes immune suppressing treatments for ILD. The biggest complaint of an ILD patient is breathlessness. Any activity that requires them to move, however mild, takes a lot of effort and leaves them short of breath. With standard treatment, there is relief from breathlessness and the disease progression does abate, but the patient's quality of life continues to be less than ideal. They have to deal with lifelong acid reflux, bloating and disturbed rest because of sleep apnoea. Loss of appetite and muscle tissue is seen in most ILD patients. The typical ILD patient appears overtly malnourished and gasping for air.

As expected, the only thing done in allopathy to improve the quality of life of an ILD patient is pharmacotherapy. One of my colleagues even lamented once that he has no idea how to make the patients comfortable aside from prescribing antacids.

The issue with the digestion of an ILD patient is primarily reflux rather than acid overproduction. What antacids do is reduce acid production. Even though that may give the patient relief for the day, it comes with its own hidden cost. The acid in our stomachs is produced for a reason. It kills the germs hiding in our food and activates pathways for protein digestion and absorption. If acid production is stopped indiscriminately, the muscle wasting problem is aggravated. With their appetite gone out the window, poor absorption from their restricted diet worsens the patient's condition.

Unani and Ayurveda recognized the plight of the ILD patient long before Western medicine. There is a whole treatment plan for ILD; I even found a few studies detailing the procedures done for these patients at an Ayurvedic retreat.[32] I will not advise you to toss all your meds out the window and go for such a retreat. But what I *can* confidently suggest is the diet advised by these two disciplines, aimed at boosting your quality of life. The underlying principles for both are the same. The diet recommended to an ILD patient would include:

1. **Cooked, easy to digest foods.** I cannot stress the importance of cooking your food enough. There is no doubt that raw vegetables retain their nutrient content. However, they are harder to digest and can exacerbate symptoms such as bloating, cramping or diarrhoea. On reaching the colon, undigested food is acted upon by bacteria and its digestion releases a lot of gas. This adds to bloating. Cooked vegetables are easier to digest. Additionally, the bioavailability of nutrients is often lower in uncooked foods. Cooking can break down tough cell walls and make nutrients more accessible to our gut for absorption.
2. **A warning to stay clear of gut irritants.** Plants may be quiet and stationary but they are not defenceless. And that defence is to preserve their nutrients for their next generation and not for you and me to eat.

A seed is programmed to conserve its nutrients for its baby. The enzymes needed to release these nutrients are activated in the presence of water. When it is soaked, the seed realizes that it's time to germinate. The same machinery which was protecting the nutrients gets unlocked. Essentially, we humans are tricking the plant into believing that it's going to live and grow. The compounds in the seed that protect it from being digested are reduced on soaking and are now bioavailable to the human eating it. If the grain is consumed unsoaked and unsprouted, those same compounds irritate the gut. Long story short: sprout, mill and cook your grains!

3. **Plenty of spice.** Incorporate warming spices into your meals to stimulate digestion and add flavour. The patient can safely consume ginger, cinnamon, cardamom, cumin, coriander, cloves and black pepper without worsening acid reflux. These spices help kindle the digestion (Agni in Ayurveda-speak) and improve nutrient absorption.
4. **Healthy fats.** Include healthy fats in your diet to counteract Vata's dryness. Opt for sources such as ghee, coconut oil, olive oil, sesame oil, nuts and seeds. These fats provide lubrication, nourishment and grounding energy.

Fermented Foods and Kapha Dosha

Fermented foods have a dual relationship to Kapha dosha, depending on their intensity and the individual's state of balance. When Kapha is stable, mild fermented foods – such as lightly cultured yogurt, homemade kanji or small amounts of pickled vegetables – can be beneficial. They act as natural prebiotics, nourishing the gut microbiota, enhancing nutrient absorption and strengthening the mucosal lining of the digestive tract. This aligns with Kapha's grounding and stabilizing qualities, supporting immunity and maintaining healthy tissue lubrication. In Ayurveda, the sour taste (amla rasa) found in fermented foods is considered mildly stimulating for digestion and can help counter Kapha's tendency towards sluggishness when used in moderation.

However, in cases of Kapha aggravation – marked by excess mucus, heaviness, congestion or fluid retention – fermented foods, particularly those that are strongly aged or preserved, can become a problem. These include aged cheese, kombucha, vinegar-based pickles and fermented soy. Biomedically, these foods are often high in histamine and other amines, which can overwhelm histamine breakdown pathways (such as the DAO enzyme), especially if gut integrity is compromised. This can lead to symptoms like acid reflux, bloating, coughing or increased mucus production as seen in sinusitis or bronchitis. Heavily fermented or sour foods should be limited when Kapha is elevated to avoid worsening inflammation and respiratory or digestive congestion. I will delve deeper into this concept in the chapter on cold foods.

6

UNDERSTANDING RITUCHARYA: THE PRINCIPLES OF SEASONAL LIVING

It is common knowledge that our bodies are around 70 per cent water. But if a branch of alternative medicine says the same in the form of humour or dosha predominance, our allopathic sensibilities find it absurd. There are times in the year when specific doshas or bio-energies predominate. Your own temperament oscillates – between hot and dry, hot and wet, cold and dry, cold and wet – as does your food's. Our body is not a machine that simply accepts food as it is. It interacts with food just as the food interacts with our body. This triad of body, food and surroundings makes each of us unique; incapable of being put into the restrictive boxes that characterize allopathic medicine. What works for the typical subject of research studies – a white male weighing 80 kg – will definitely not reflect in the same way on a 60 kg brown female.

As the seasons change, so does the body: from the microscopic bacteria living in your mouth to oil production in your skin to the raging appetite that awakens with the cold. The natural rhythms of your body control your sleep-wake cycle, periods, stress responses – everything ebbs and flows. Throughout the year our bodies follow the old adage that change is the only constant.

The variations in the body's reaction to the changing seasons are especially noticeable when it comes to gender. For example, research shows that males and females differ in both body temperature rhythms and reactions to atmospheric heat.[33] Body temperature in spring and summer is higher for females, while males adapt to the surrounding heat due to a dip in their metabolism. Another study found a noted decrease in plasma levels of TSH in males in hot, dry conditions. Females showed no difference in thyroid function in hot, dry conditions despite their bodies adapting to the stress of changing weather conditions.

Ritucharya is an essential concept in Ayurveda that means 'seasonal regimen' (*ritu*: season, *charya*: routine). It is based on the understanding that the human body is deeply connected to nature and its internal balance necessarily aligns with external changes. Ayurveda recognizes six seasons, each influencing the balance of the three doshas. Food, lifestyle and behaviour in each season must adapt to support digestion (Agni), immunity (*Ojas*) and mental clarity (*Sattva*). The core principle is that like increases like, while the opposite brings balance.

In these guidelines I will speak in terms of doshas due to the lack of sufficient scientific vocabulary. When I mention that a particular dosha is imbalanced, it is usually not within its ideal range. For instance, thyroid function is higher in the winter and lower in the summer, while central sensitivity (the Pitta effect) to thyroid hormones increases in the summer and decreases in the winter. So, when it is said that Pitta 'increases' in the summer, it translates to the body's hormetic balance being disturbed. Some people are more prone to certain imbalances depending on their body's inherent temperament.

Hemanta (Early Winter) and Shishira (Late Winter)

Mid-November to Mid-March
Dominant dosha: Kapha begins accumulating

In these cold months, the body can handle richer, heavier foods. This is the ideal time to nourish and build strength.

- Have warm, oily, nourishing meals that include ghee, whole milk, soup, meat broth, urad dal, sesame, nuts and root vegetables (sweet potato, carrot, beetroot). Use warming spices such as ginger, black pepper, cinnamon and mustard seeds.
- Avoid cold, raw or light foods like salads or smoothies.
- Have a warm breakfast complete with ghee and grains. Lunch should be your heaviest meal. Enjoy

warm milk mixed with nutmeg or turmeric at night to support deep rest.

Vasanta (Spring)

Mid-March to Mid-May
Dominant dosha: Kapha aggravates

In spring, the body may naturally feel heavier and more sluggish, mirroring what Ayurveda calls Kapha accumulation. This can show up as slower digestion, mild fluid retention, congestion or seasonal allergies. These effects happen because of environmental changes like humidity, pollen and temperature shifts which influence metabolism, immune response and mucus production. Warmer weather has a mucolytic (mucus thinning) effect, linked to allergies and seasonal conjunctivitis. The focus is now on detoxification and lightening the system.

- Prioritize light, dry and warm foods like barley, millets, lentils, steamed vegetables and light soups. Spices such as trikatu (a classic Ayurvedic blend of dry ginger, black pepper and pippali) and turmeric help improve digestion.
- Avoid dairy, oily foods, heavy grains, cold drinks and sweets.
- Begin the day with warm water infused with honey and lemon. The bitter of the lemon rind and mucolytic action of honey help combat allergic predisposition. Emphasize astringent, bitter and pungent tastes to reduce excess Kapha.

Grishma (Summer)

Mid-May to Mid-July
Dominant dosha: Pitta accumulates

During this intensely hot and dry season, Pitta starts increasing and digestive fire weakens due to external heat. The goal is to keep cool, hydrated and avoid overstimulation.

- Consume sweet, cooling and hydrating foods like cucumber, melons, coconut water, rose water, rice, milk and ghee. Cooling herbs include coriander, fennel and mint. These foods help reduce the heat generated by increased central sensitivity to the thyroid hormone.
- Avoid spicy, sour, fermented or salty foods, along with excessive exertion or heat-producing activities.
- Eat small, frequent meals. Drink infusions like coriander-fennel tea. Try not to skip meals but keep your food light and refreshing.

Varsha (Monsoon)

Mid-July to Mid-September
Dominant dosha: Vata aggravates, Agni weakens

The rainy season showers our bodies with dampness, digestive irregularities and increased susceptibility to infections. With Vata on the rise, the priority is to stabilize digestion and prevent imbalances.

- Go for warm, light and slightly oily foods like khichdi, rice, moong dal and soups. Favour ginger, cumin and asafoetida while tempering your dishes to kindle digestion and reduce gas buildup. These foods and spices have prebiotic and carminative properties that reduce the Vata imbalance, improve digestion and prevent bloating.
- Avoid leafy greens, raw salads, curd and cold beverages, as they increase dampness and disturb Agni.
- Sip warm water through the day. Consume ghee to nourish your tissues without clogging digestion. Avoid heavy outdoor activity and ensure rest.

Sharad (Autumn)

Mid-September to Mid-November
Dominant dosha: Pitta aggravates

Autumn, though cool, is dry and sharp, further aggravating Pitta. After the summer heat, Pitta peaks in this season. Cooling, mildly sweet and bitter foods can help pacify it.

- Eat light and cooling items such as basmati rice, amla, pomegranate, bitter gourd and cooked greens. Use cooling spices like coriander, fennel and cardamom.
- Avoid hot, spicy and oily foods, as well as items that are excessively fermented or acidic.
- Have your meals on time and avoid fasting. Begin the day with pomegranate. Apply coconut oil or sandalwood to your skin and hair for cooling.

Personalizing Ritucharya

In Ayurveda, the optimal seasonal routine of Ritucharya is further refined by adapting it to the individual's prakruti (constitution). The questionnaire at the end of Chapter 1 would have allowed you to find out more about your prakruti.

Vata Predominant Individuals

- **Winter:** This is a stabilizing season for Vata. Embrace warming, heavy and oily foods. Milk, ghee, urad dal, sesame and wheat are beneficial.
- **Spring:** Vata stays balanced but can feel scattered. Favour warm, spiced and grounding meals. Avoid cold salads.
- **Summer:** Heat can dehydrate Vata. Juicy, cooling, moist foods like watermelon, coconut water and rice are helpful.
- **Monsoon:** This is the worst season for Vata. Digestion is weak. Eat ginger, asafoetida, moong dal and soups in plenty. Avoid dry beans and raw food.
- **Autumn:** Can be destabilizing for Vata. Consume slightly sweet, bitter and grounding foods like cooked rice, bottle gourd and cow's milk.
- Gentle grounding practices like yoga, tai chi, walking or light swimming are ideal for the Vata predominant. Shorter sessions of exercise (between twenty to thirty minutes) four to five days a week work well.
- Avoid overstimulation and irregular routines.

Pitta Predominant Individuals

- **Winter:** Enjoy richer foods but in moderation. Use ghee, barley, wheat and milk.
- **Spring:** Pitta is naturally balanced. Favour light, bitter foods like green vegetables – especially bitter gourd – and lentils.
- **Summer:** The worst season for Pitta. Eat cooling, hydrating foods such as cucumber, coconut, rose and pomegranate. Avoid spicy or oily foods.
- **Monsoon:** Pitta can be slightly aggravated. Use digestive spices like cumin and fennel. Avoid fermented, sour food.
- **Autumn:** Pitta peaks. Focus on bitter and sweet tastes: amla, coriander, neem and rice. Avoid chili, mustard and alcohol.
- Try cooling, non-competitive forms of exercise like swimming, cycling in the morning, calming yoga and walks in nature. Thirty to forty-five-minute-long sessions five times a week are optimal. Avoid midday heat and overexertion.

Kapha Predominant Individuals

- **Winter:** Kapha begins accumulating. Eat light, spicy, dry foods like barley, millets, lentils and warm soups.
- **Spring:** The worst season for Kapha. Detox with bitter and pungent tastes. Use ginger, trikatu and turmeric. Avoid dairy.
- **Summer:** Favour fresh fruits, bitter greens and light grains. Avoid overeating and dairy.

- **Monsoon:** Digestion is weak but Kapha remains stable. Prioritize warm, light food. Avoid raw and cold food.
- **Autumn:** A good time to strengthen immunity. Choose warming but not oily foods. Avoid sugary and fried items.
- Kapha types benefit most from intensive workouts like cardio, dancing, jogging, fast-paced yoga or resistance training. Exercise daily or at least five to six times a week for forty minutes to an hour. Morning is the best time to work out and stimulate sluggish energy.

7

YOUR BODY IN THE WINTER

The Sanskrit medical texts *Charaka Samhita* and *Ashtanga Hridayam* both outline how to balance your body's temperament in the winter season. As per Ayurveda, the arrival of winter is accompanied by the withdrawal of Agni into the body. In more scientific terms, our blood is redistributed to the core of the body to maintain surface and core temperature within a normal range. The blood from our limbs is shuttled to our internal organs, contributing to slightly higher BP in the winter. A simple example of this redistribution is your toenails turning blue when temperatures drop to the single digits.

Ayurvedic wisdom suggests that there is a corresponding increase in digestive fire due to the inward movement of Agni. Contemporary researchers have observed a similar pattern in our digestive processes. Studies have shown that stomach ulcers are more common in cold climates than hot ones. Infection by the ulcer-causing bacteria *H. pylori* was also found to be a lot more common in subjects living in colder climates.[34] The lower the temperature, the higher the chance of complications like bleeding or perforation of gut ulcers. In fact, it is also impacted by the degree of temperature variation. The stomach has a protective mucus layer that prevents stomach acid from digesting the organ itself – yes, kind of freaky to imagine. This mucus lining is thinner in the winter than summer.

When we consume protein, it is gradually broken down into smaller parts called amino acids. These amino acids travel through the body and are reassembled by different cells to make the proteins they need. In winter, this process slows down because of seasonal changes in our genes. Certain genes that drive repair, growth and immunity switch to a lower gear, while others that conserve energy or store fat become more active. This seasonal 'reprogramming' is nature's way of slowing down so that the body can focus on survival and the conservation of resources. As a result, the protective protein layer in the stomach lining becomes thinner. This means the gut is more vulnerable during the colder months and we should support it by eating foods that are gentle and easy to digest. Additionally, certain proteins that function as supervisors for the smooth running of cells (for example, heat shock proteins) are produced at a lower rate in the biting cold.

With regard to tissue function, the immune system has a pro-inflammatory function during winter. The blood markers of heart disease risk, psychiatric illnesses and autoimmune diseases (wherein your immune system attacks the body itself) are at peak levels in winter. Our vitamin D receptors also increase in the summer months and decrease in winter. Since sunlight exposure is limited during colder months, the body must work with what little it gets. Having a bit more body fat can be beneficial in this context, as it helps absorb and transport fat-soluble vitamins like D and K, both of which are crucial for bone health. In turn, this enhances calcium uptake from dietary sources, supporting skeletal strength despite reduced sun exposure.

Cold weather can exacerbate arthritis, a condition that causes joint pain, swelling and limitation of movement. There are many causes of arthritis but the most common kinds – osteoarthritis and rheumatoid – generally worsen in winter. Unfortunately, the winter season is a nightmare for those with musculoskeletal issues, be it arthritis, autoimmune diseases or just creaky joints. This is due in part to an increase in muscle spasming around joints and a decrease in blood circulation. In patients with rheumatoid arthritis, lower disease activity is observed when there is more sunshine and low humidity.

The production of the stress hormone cortisol is reduced during winter; however, blood levels of cortisol increase and our tissues are more sensitive to its action. This contributes to the increased prevalence of disease during this season. Higher winter cortisol reshapes immunity, metabolism, mood, cardiovascular stress, gut function and sleep, making the body more pro-inflammatory, infection-prone, mood-vulnerable and metabolically stressed. The lack of light in the winter can give rise to a psychiatric condition called Seasonal Affective Disorder (or SAD) that leaves you feeling just that – sad. This depressive disorder affects people in winter, leaving them moody, cranky and generally low on energy. As I lead you through warming and hot foods that are best suited for those cold months, I will share examples of how to eat better to stabilize the winter blues.

Starting Your Winter Diet

I take issue with the concept of a static balanced diet where every calorie must be perfectly accounted for. Despite the modern obsession with restrictive eating, we are so far from being as healthy as our ancestors. Come hail or snow, Instagram influencers demand that our plates should be a mosaic of avocado green and cherry tomato red, topped with the sheen of salad dressing. Breakfast smoothies packed with bananas, blueberries and protein powder are necessary to kickstart your day – nutrients packed into a mason jar. But that begs the question, how can your plate look the same all year round when neither your body nor the environment remain constant? Your gut bacteria, body clock, every cell of your body – all of them change and adapt. It's time that we take a hard look at what we are putting into our bodies. Do we really need that much greenery to chug and chew? Or should we respect the tenets of eating seasonally and provide our body with the nourishment it needs rather than copy-paste a formula which is failing millions around the world?

For instance, since our immunity tends to go down during the winter, we are pressed to consume vitamin C to boost it. Vitamin C is great, yes. But is it the be-all and end-all of immunity? Absolutely not. Fruit and vegetable smoothies are great theoretically but have practical limitations in the winter. The gut is weaker in the cold season and has to work that much harder to digest uncooked foods, even if they are pureed into oblivion! Cooking initiates the digestion process on the stove itself and is far kinder to our gut. That does not mean we have to cook fruits and never eat dry fruits. But the salad-smoothie craze is costing us much more than just our ease of digestion; it is causing us actual harm.

It is 100 per cent true that vitamin C does not get stored in our bodies like other fat-soluble vitamins. However, it does get converted into a chemical called oxalate that can get deposited in your kidneys in the form of calcium oxalate stones. The downpour of nutrients in juice form might actually clog up your kidneys. People usually megadose vitamin C for immunity, faster recovery from infections, skin brightening, surgery healing, fitness recovery, unsubstantiated cancer reversal or because of wellness trends promoting high antioxidant intake. These practices can easily push intake above 2–4 g a day – the range where oxalate production begins to rise. There have been cases where people have suffered acute kidney failure because of juice cleanses – ironically often marketed as a way to 'flush toxins'![35,36] A heavy price to pay for glowing skin.

There is remarkable evidence that our body's good bacteria not only respond to cold stress but also affect heat production in our bodies. You need to take care of these little guys by maintaining a good diet. Short-chain fatty acids (SCFAs) like acetate and butyrate are produced by the action of good gut bacteria on the food we eat. These SCFAs help produce body heat and reduce the inflammation that occurs during winter. Our increased appetite in the colder months is not only to cushion our body but also provide more food to our hungry gut bacteria to fight the biting chill. Butyrate also protects the intestine by coating it and preventing a leaky gut. This means better digestion, better motions and a happier gut.

Research shows that mammals without gut microbes – either under lab conditions or soon after using antibiotics – have lower body temperatures and struggle more in the cold.[37,38] The bacteria present in our gut help our body harvest heat-producing molecules and maintain a normal core temperature regardless of the chill outside (remember homeostasis?). Directly introducing the energy-packed SCFAs produced by bacteria into the intestine provided added protection from cold stress. It is also important to note that eating high-fibre foods helps sustain these bacteria. The gut bacteria act upon the fibre and ferment it as it passes along our digestive system. The heat generated by this fermentation process accounts for about three-fourth of our body's heat production.

Fresh veggies that we consume in the summer are better digested by the population of *Bacteroides* in our gut. The Bacteroidetes species specializes in degrading high molecular weight organic material such as plant cell walls and complex carbohydrates. These bacteria protect us from bloating and indigestion caused by consuming too much fibre in the form of fresh fruits and vegetables. Come winter, their numbers start to go down. The relative abundance of this species in our gut during the summer and the drop during winter is consistent with the wisdom of eating more fruits and vegetables in the warmer season.

The temperature of food also makes a difference. A chilled smoothie or tossed salad affects the airways by stimulating the temperature receptors in our internal organs. This causes increased mucus secretion and constriction of the airways, adding to airway hyperreactivity – think wheezing and coughing up phlegm. So much for salads increasing immunity! Apart from affecting our airways, the cold temperature of food also affects the gut function. Warm foods relax the stomach and intestine whereas cold foods cause contraction. A relaxed gut means less gas build-up as gas escapes from the colon easily, giving us bloat-free winters.

All in all, don't fall for this smoothie and that salad being promoted by your calorie-counting app. It is quite difficult to harvest the goodness of out-of-season vegetables. And you will only be able to prevent that bloat during winter if you steer clear of salads and particularly smoothies.

Avoid drying, pungent and astringent foods and go for sweet and savoury flavours. Warming, heavy foods are what both your common sense and gut will tell you to have in the winter. Cook and steam your food to reduce its starch content, easing digestion and absorption. Slow cooking goat trotters (*paaya*) helps extract minerals and gelatin from the bone. Warm, delicious and a powerhouse of minerals, this soup is the perfect comfort drink.

With the digestive system being in an active phase in the winter, nutritional strengthening of the gut is generally more helpful than in other seasons. As per traditional medicine, the intake of oily foods should be increased during winter. Enter ghee, the nation's favourite fat. Indian festivals go hand in hand with ghee-laden sweets. Thank God that our fattening festivals fall in the winter, when our increased appetite serves a greater purpose. The goodness of ghee during this season is unparalleled. It nourishes your body – and especially your gut – like no other source of fat can. It is a great prebiotic, takes good care of your gut bacteria and decreases acidity in the stomach. Also, it is an excellent medium for transporting fat-soluble vitamins to our tissues.

The King of All Fats

Ghee is the master of all trades. A warm food by nature with a cooling effect on the gut, it is not an exception to the rule but a rule in itself.

One of the basic principles of ghee consumption is to have it in the afternoon. Ayurveda tells us that ghee balances the fire in the body. Though this might sound cuckoo to our ears, it abounds in wisdom. For food to be consumed, energy must be spent in its digestion and absorption. This is called the 'thermic effect' of food. Thermic effect adds to the metabolic rate of the person, which means the heat production in the body is increased and calories are spent. It varies from morning to evening, following the body's natural rhythm. Ghee does not significantly elevate this thermic effect, unlike protein- or carbohydrate-rich foods, since fats require less energy to digest and metabolize. This is why the sages tried to tell us about ghee calming the Pitta (fire) of the body. The body's core temperature is highest in the evening, due to its internal rhythm. Lunch with a serving of ghee helps balance out this core temperature fluctuation by the time evening sets in.

The medium-chain fatty acids (MCFAs) of ghee help burn fat, keep our metabolic rates stable in winter and protect us from metabolic diseases like high cholesterol and diabetes. Ghee also contains butyric acid – the same SCFA that your healthy gut bacteria produce from fibre. Even if we do consume an adequate amount of fibre, our gut is often not healthy enough to produce butyrate from it. So, ghee is practically serving butyrate to your bacteria on a platter!

Let's consider other parts of our food tract. Starting from the stomach, ghee reduces ulcer formation and offers relief from bloating and gastritis. The liver is the next to benefit. Just a gentle reminder: Vata dosha, the master of transport and communication in the body, tends to go a bit haywire in the winter. That's where ghee comes to the rescue. It supports bile flow, boosts motility in the biliary ducts and promotes cholesterol excretion – all of which help keep gallstones at bay. These good fats also aid in fat digestion and keep cholesterol in check. This becomes especially relevant for women over forty, who are more prone to gallstones. Medical professionals cheekily sum up the risk factors with a mnemonic: 'fat, fertile female of forty'.

Next, we enter the intestinal zone where the real action happens. Butyrate regulates fluid transport across the intestinal barrier and reduces mucosal inflammation caused due to poor dietary habits or bad bacteria. The butyrate from ghee also reinforces the defence barrier of the intestine, making it less permeable to toxins. The cherry on top is that the butyric acid from ghee helps remove damaged cells and mitigates inflammation, protecting us from colorectal cancer.

Mitochondrial Function in the Winter

One of the primary roles of mitochondria is thermogenesis, the process of generating heat to maintain body temperature. The need for sources of fat in the winter is manifold. The most well-known of our defences against cold weather is shivering. Another less-discussed mechanism is the brown fat in our body. Though very important for babies, as we grow older, brown fat is replaced by white fat – the kind we sweat in the gym to get rid of!

Now, between the two kinds of fat, lies 'beige fat'. It forms when certain cells in white fat start taking on the characteristics of brown fat, like having more mitochondria and burning energy to produce heat. Also known as 'brite' (brown-in-white) fat, it is an important part of the body's thermostat. In winter, cold exposure activates brown fat mitochondria to produce heat, increasing energy expenditure. Hormones like norepinephrine trigger this response and stimulate the formation of new mitochondria, especially in the muscles, improving overall metabolic health.

While excess unhealthy fats can damage mitochondrial function, certain fats are beneficial for mitochondrial health. Ghee and edible oils contain essential fatty acids and antioxidants that protect the mitochondria. Ghee might be the king of all fats but he has a few noble ministers in his court.

1. **Olive Oil**: A staple of the Mediterranean diet, olive oil is rich in monounsaturated fats and polyphenols. These are potent antioxidants that help maintain mitochondrial health. Studies have shown that diets that are high in olive oil improve mitochondrial biogenesis, the process by which new mitochondria are formed, thus enhancing energy metabolism. Disclaimer: Do not overuse it or replace your native oils!
2. **Coconut Oil**: It is rich in medium-chain triglycerides (MCTs), which are metabolized differently than other fats. MCTs are rapidly absorbed and transported directly to the liver, where they are converted into ketones. Ketones are an alternative energy source for mitochondria and can improve mitochondrial efficiency, especially in conditions of metabolic stress. Ketones also reduce the production of oxidants and enhance mitochondrial function.

This is just tip of the iceberg of healthy fats. I deal with oil and cholesterol at length in Chapter Eleven.

Spices: Hot, Hot Baby!

Not all spices are made equal. Black pepper, saffron and turmeric are all considered 'hot' spices, yet each represents a distinct style of warmth. Black pepper, along with other pungent spices like chili and ginger, carries a sharp, energizing heat that stimulates digestion and circulation. Turmeric, like cumin or mustard, provides gentler, nourishing warmth that supports the liver and reduces inflammation. Saffron, alongside aromatic spices such as cinnamon and cardamom, offers a subtle, fragrant heat that uplifts one's mood. Together, the trio exhibits the range of 'hot' qualities in spices, from intense and stimulating to gentle and restorative.

Black pepper – the anti-bloat spice

Spices almost always have a hot nature – coriander seeds, saunf and soaked methi being exceptions. The way they are described in traditional medicine, their effect on our taste buds, the sweating they can cause – every aspect of spices shouts hot. For both their observable effects and subtle physiological impact, these tiny doses of goodness in food have earned the label of hot foods.

Hot foods are inherently programmed to evacuate clogged up waste from the body. When the Vata dosha goes awry in winter, it can be balanced using foods which maintain the plumbing of our body, be it gaseous waste causing bloating or irregular periods. Spices improve kidney function to increase urine excretion (diuretic action) and improve bowel movements (laxative action). They also cause sweating (diaphoretic action) and clear out the skin. The compounds present in black pepper improve kidney filtration, conduction through nerves and liver function. When our bodies seasonally go into fat-storing mode, this spice – and many others – open the blood vessels to the internal organs, improve nerve function and ensure we don't move towards developing metabolic diseases by storing fat in the wrong places.

Black pepper is used in kitchens everywhere to add zing to bland dishes and even introduce young children to Indian spices. In Indian cuisine, black pepper is used in a variety of hot dishes that are ready to burn your palate in the most fun way possible: kali mirch chicken and pepper liver fry to name a few. Biryani – be it Bengali, Lucknowi or Hyderabadi – is incomplete without whole spices in the rice and ground spices in the biryani masala, both of which often include black pepper. And how can we forget black pepper mixed with honey as a home remedy for the common cold and cough?

Allergies are caused by hyperactive airway inflammation. The beauty of the Indian spice box is that it neither suppresses the immune system like pharma drugs nor does it let your body run amok. Spices have this amazing ability to modulate your immune system. In particular, turmeric and black pepper have emerged as fantastic immunomodulators in recent studies.[39] Pepper suppresses nasal itchiness, reduces inflammation in the nasal passage and helps minimize sneezing. The active compound in pepper, piperine, decreases the influx of allergy cells into the nasal mucous surface. The action of pepper extends all the way to the endpoint of the airways – the alveoli – where it reduces airway hyperresponsiveness and chest congestion.

Spices have a wonderful carminative effect, i.e., they help remove gas build-up, relieving bloating. And if you notice, heavy non-vegetarian foods (think Hyderabadi Haleem or Biryani) have a lovely flavour layup in each morsel. The spices facilitate digestion by improving circulation to the digestive tract, increasing the secretion of digestive juices and slowing gastric emptying. The gradual emptying of food increases nutrient absorption and ensures you are satisfied for longer, which helps cut back calories in the long run.

Pepper has a special place in the life of a diabetic. It inhibits liver enzymes to make diabetes medication more available to the body and its direct effect on intestinal cells promotes drug absorption. Black pepper also reduces bad cholesterol and increases good cholesterol. It prevents fat accumulation and plaque build-up in the arteries by inhibiting certain enzymes. It aids in reversing insulin resistance and helps manage diabetes and Polycystic Ovary Syndrome (PCOS).

Some antidepressants in the market fall under the compound category of monoamine oxidase inhibitors. They inhibit a specific enzyme in the brain, thus allowing happy hormones to remain in your system for longer and keep your spirits up. Piperine shows similar properties. Winter months tend to negatively affect our mood. Both SAD and pre-existing mental illnesses are likely to flare up during the colder months. Adding a pinch of pepper to a warm broth and comforting foods might ease you somewhat during this time.

Another hot property of pepper is that it causes sweating. Its active compounds increase blood flow to the skin, making it flush. So, if someone asks you why we Indians gorge on these spices, just tell them they're our natural highlighters!

But it is oh so easy to overshoot. Such is the post-Industrial Revolution world. If we see a good thing, our instinct is to extrapolate the hell out of it. Think of vitamin C. It's important; it saved sailors from scurvy. So, of course, we have pilled it up and lapped it up. Pills? Check! Fortified yeast? Double check! Oil and ghee? Check! Capsicum and potato and orange, the natural sources of vitamin C? Not so much. Then you have fat on the other hand. For years, there was an outcry of 'Fat is bad for the heart!' or 'Ban it!' If you ask me, fat was the first victim of cancel culture even before cancel culture was a thing. Now a few decades later, we've come around to 'Good fat is good for the heart!'

Pretty much the same thing happened to our spices during the Covid-immunity-boosting frenzy. Find me one Indian who has not received a WhatsApp forward making tall claims about a *kadha* and I will show you someone who lives under a rock. A kadha is a medicinal home remedy made by boiling spices in water. There is no one recipe; in fact, there are many kinds of kadha for different conditions. Here is a simple recipe for a kadha for treating a cold:

Boil a few cloves, black peppercorns, 1 inch of ginger and a handful of tulsi leaves in one cup of water for ten minutes. Allow the mixture to cool. Strain and serve with some honey.

You might notice that all the spices and herbs in this are of a hot nature. Even the sweetening agent, honey, is hot.

Kadha is recommended during acute viral illnesses in small measures (twenty to thirty millilitres). In no form does it boost immunity if consumed daily in larger quantities. Pepper and other spices may work as immunomodulators but the sky is *not* the limit when it comes to immunity boosting. We all should have resisted the temptation of extrapolation during that time. In fact, many Ayurvedic doctors as well as the Ministry of Ayush urged the public to not drink kadha more than twice a day and that too in limited quantities. The fact of the matter is that kadhas might have been helpful during Covid or Covid-like illnesses because the concoction has a virus binding effect and helps in faster recovery. However, this wonderful home remedy was exploited to such an extreme that the humble kadha ended up hurting us.

In my own practice I saw patients suffering from gastritis and heartburn because of overconsumption of kadha. The same pepper which was supposed to help them tread a middle path was heating their insides like a furnace. And it didn't stop at that. One of my colleagues, an eye doctor, told me that he has been seeing so many more case of uveitis ever since the kadha craze caught on. Uveitis is the inflammation of the middle layer of the eye, resulting in redness and a burning sensation. Though reversible, it can turn chronic and compromise vision. Unfortunately, we were unable to find any papers citing a rise in cases of uveitis due to kadha.

A quick Google search and you will be flooded with

recipes that are presented as the magic cure that will halt diabetes, somehow burn the stubborn fat around your organs, shave off those extra kilos, stop heart disease in its tracks and basically alter your life. Online sources have come up with dozens of ways to consume the humble pepper. Most will be along the lines of: chew it or drink black pepper tea first thing in the morning to melt fat away. Your body fat is not refrigerated butter. So no, it shall not melt.

Be cautious that all claims are tall claims. For instance, I mentioned that diabetics may stand to benefit from black pepper. That's where moderation comes in. If you consume black pepper in excess, on an empty stomach or worse, take pepper supplements as a way to shed those pounds and singlehandedly battle diabetes, you are in for a rude but expected shock. It ain't a magic pill.

Every single thing on this planet is a chemical. The water you drink is hydrogen oxide. The salt, sodium chloride. In the same vein, black pepper is also a chemical – well, lots of awesome chemicals bundled up neatly into a tiny, fragrant ball. These chemicals interact on a cellular level with our body's enzymes and slowly yet surely can give rise to side effects. If you overdose on it, the side effects will be much sooner to follow.

For people who have bleeding disorders or are on blood thinners, excess pepper consumption can lead to prolonged bleeding time. The same mechanism of delayed clotting can increase menstrual blood flow. Too much black pepper can irritate the stomach and intestinal lining, potentially causing painful ulcers. This aligns with Ayurveda's idea of black pepper being a *pramathi* spice, which means it 'scrapes' the intestines – not literally like a brush but by helping shed old cells. Since intestinal cells multiply quickly, there's a higher risk of mutation, which can lead to cancer if left unchecked. Black pepper helps trigger the natural death of these fast-growing cells, preventing rogue cells from sticking around too long and making it a powerful protector against cancer.

You might feel like we are back to square one. Confused as to how you can incorporate this special yet seemingly dangerous spice into your diet? Avoid extremes and eat the spice how a spice should be eaten: in very little quantities. Think of spice as a *chhota* packet, *bada* punch.

1. Add whole peppercorns to your tadkas, especially when making non-vegetarian gravies.
2. Use it in the garam masala you finish your dishes with to add zing to your meals.
3. When down with a viral, sip on a warm homemade kadha. Don't make it a Venti order! Fifteen to thirty millilitres twice a day is enough.
4. Sprinkle black pepper powder on boiled eggs or warm broths on chilly days.
5. Sprinkle the powder on sweet fruits to add flavour and negate their cold effect.
6. Make it a point to consume more pepper in the winter than summer.

Turmeric – the immunity modulator

Haldi is present in all aspects of Indian life from the cradle to the grave. Newborn babies are bathed with ubtan – usually made with besan (chickpea flour), a smaller quantity of another flour (jowar or rice) and a pinch of the healing turmeric. The turmeric in the ubtan prevents bacteria from sticking to the baby's skin. In the growing-up years, moms apply turmeric on scrapes and wounds. In sickness, haldi milk is our saviour whereas in health, our foods are incomplete without the deep tint of yellow that the West generalizes as curry-coloured. Those who practise the Hindu faith hold haldi in great esteem and use it in religious ceremonies. The bride and groom are smeared with turmeric before their wedding day and this fun tradition is called, you guessed it, the haldi ceremony! Come old age you are popping curcumin pills (a very new addition to the Indian lifestyle) and smearing turmeric-tinged balms on your achy knees.

Like most spices, turmeric is a hot food. We usually cannot feel its heating effects because of how little we consume on a daily basis. But even a humble pinch of haldi offers so many benefits for the whole body. What if I told you haldi protects you from heart disease due to its blood thinning effect? That it reduces chronic inflammation – the same chronic inflammation that can lead to diabetes and high cholesterol levels; that can put you at risk of cancer in practically any part of the body.

Turmeric's best effects are documented in the gut, since the two come in direct contact. It also protects the mouth, salivary glands and food pipe from cancer. It has antibacterial properties that work against the stomach cancer-causing bacteria *Helicobacter pylori*. Regular consumption reduces liver ailments caused due to hepatitis C, fat in the liver and excess alcohol consumption. In cancer research, curcumin (the active ingredient in haldi) is emerging as a strong contender for cancer chemotherapy of intestinal tumours because it can suppress cancer-growth pathways directly in the gut, where it achieves higher local concentrations with minimal systemic toxicity. Very little curcumin is absorbed into the bloodstream, so most of it stays inside the gut – right where intestinal tumours form. It also has a beneficial effect on celiac disease (gluten intolerance) and inflammatory bowel disease.

Even though turmeric stands out as an anti-cancer drug – with remarkable inhibition of breast, prostate and blood cancer – its bioavailability is limited. Pepper increases its absorption and retention in the body, making them great to have together. In fact, adding a pinch of pepper in your haldi *ka doodh* can improve the absorption of turmeric by a whopping 200 per cent! Be it in your cooking or turmeric-pepper milk, this *jodi* is made in the heavens.

What would you do upon hearing about these miracles brought about by this taken-for-granted spice? Perhaps drink it up, pop it as a pill, gulp down the curries ... sniff it, snort it, directly inject it into your veins?

Well, that is kind of what the West has done after discovering the active ingredient of turmeric, curcumin. It has been extracted, purified and marketed as curcumin supplements. You don't need a prescription to pop a haldi pill – just walk to the nearest health store. In the US, next to the stacks and stacks of protein powder and steroids disguised as muscle food, you can find a nice supply of this wonder drug. Haldi is being sold in the US for around ₹450 a kilogram, when the same costs ₹70 in India. Starbucks in now marketing overpriced haldi ka doodh while influencers use it as a topper for salads and eggs! I am gonna say that again: they are sprinkling haldi on eggs and raw veggies. I can't help but facepalm.

We can't blame this abuse and misuse solely on the West. For the longest time, haldi was a part of the regular Indian diet in an uncomplicated and sustainable way. Simply add a pinch to your food while cooking. No one was trying to profit off of her humble health benefits. Now the Indian public is concocting kadhas like never before and drinking them indiscriminately – irrespective of health conditions, menstrual status and without really knowing when, how and most importantly, how *much* to consume. And as expected, the side effects have begun to surface.

The dosage of curcumin supplements has not yet been standardized. Most formulations differ from one another in content and dose due to lack of FDA regulation. The reality is that the FDA doesn't really say much about health supplements, so you are gambling with your health when you take them. Some curcumin supplement formulations include pepper to increase its absorption. However, the pure form of turmeric has a narrow therapeutic window. The range between the minimum effective dose and a toxic dose is minimal, meaning slight variations can lead to ineffective treatment or toxicity. The noted side effects to date include rashes, nausea, changed stool patterns and headaches.

Curcumin also has a blood thinning effect. Taken in moderation through food it has a protective action against strokes and heart attacks. But in its pure pill form, curcumin can cause internal bleeds and further enhance the effect of blood thinning medication. When indiscriminately taken by those with liver duct problems, such supplements can increase bile production, further aggravating the issue. Not to worry though, you can safely consume turmeric in food form. The quarter teaspoon you add to a meal for a family of four is enough and will not have an adverse effect even if taken daily for the rest of your life.

Bonus, turmeric is nature's very own glow and lovely! Applying turmeric on skin promotes epithelial cell turnover (healthy baby cells surface, making your skin supple), reduces inflammation (goodbye acne and irritated skin) and modulates melanocyte activity – the cells which produce skin pigment. Curcumin slows down the enzyme tyrosinase, which makes melanin in the skin, leading to less melanin being produced. It also affects certain pathways in the skin cells involved in melanin production, helping to control melanocyte function. Thus, using turmeric on skin has been found to fade dark spots and even out skin tone.

For a homemade face pack, mix two tablespoons of besan with half a teaspoon of rice flour and a pinch of turmeric. Add water till you get a paste-like consistency. Apply over your face and wash after ten minutes. Easy!

Turmeric does not need to enter your blood directly through the gut to exert its effects. The gut benefits as it passes through and so does the skin. Turmeric has a great skin penetration, which is useful to manage joint stiffness and inflammation. In Ayurveda, turmeric *lepam* (paste) is used to treat rheumatoid and osteoarthritis. The lepam is made of fresh aloe vera and turmeric heated for few minutes and generously applied to the affected joint. The smeared area is wrapped in castor leaves to ensure the powder doesn't fall off once dry. It is left for three to five hours. This treatment helps reduce joint pain, bring down inflammation and increase the patient's range of movement.

8

WINTER STAPLES: HOT FOODS FOR THE COLD MONTHS

You don't need to install a heater in your body to tackle the winter – you need a seasonal approach to nutrition. Due to the changes we discussed in the previous chapter, our bodies require a different kind of nourishment from the warmer months. Bear in mind that the foods we eat should complement our body's changing physiology and function as well as complement one another. The quintessential Indian cooking base includes onions, ginger, garlic and often tomatoes. While onions, ginger and garlic are warming in nature, tomato is cooling. That does not mean we should completely shun the tomato in our winter cooking. Hot rasam and tomato soup will always be winter staples. Cooking changes the nature of food and regardless, we are looking to balance seasonal biological changes rather than go towards any extreme.

In the winter, Ayurveda suggests including grains with warming properties in your diet to balance the cold and damp characteristics of the environment. Wheat is warming and chapatis, parathas and daliya provide suitable nourishment during colder weather. Oats are nourishing and grounding, so oatmeal, porridge and other oat-based dishes make great breakfast options. Among the millets, ragi and bajra happen to be of a warming nature. Bajra roti is a staple in many North Indian states during winter, while ragi balls are a kannadiga classic come winter or summer. Even though rice happens to have cooling properties, it can be consumed with abandon in winter, particularly in the form of a comforting khichdi.

Functional Favourites for Winter

Since we all love shortcuts and superfoods, I will start off with functional foods that you need to include in your winter diet. The most important point to remember is that these should be consumed in small quantities. Side effects are inevitable when you cross the line and you will be forced to miss out on some fantastic, nutrient-dense foods.

Functional foods are defined broadly as foods that provide more than just nutrition – they supply specific physiological benefits to the consumer. They do not help treat disease but instead focus on prevention. Unlike foods that are fortified with vitamins, these are not used as additives. Health Canada identifies functional foods as containing bioactive principles – naturally occurring compounds that have a beneficial effect on the body.[40]

Honestly speaking, every food has a function – thus every food is a functional food. As per these outdated definitions, 'regular' foods provide only energy and proteins whereas functional foods are blessings from the heavens. In reality, all foods – from the farm to our fridge – have inherent nutritional value. There is no such thing as *just* food. Even the so-called anti-nutrients present in certain foods have a function, as do the praise-worthy phytonutrients. On the other hand, nutrient-dense foods could be causing you more harm than good if you consume them in excess in pursuit of their purported health benefits.

Nonetheless, let us dive into functional foods as defined by the nutrition media and see how they can help us better ourselves from cell to spirit.

Saffron – the anti-inflammatory in red

Saffron (*Crocus sativus*) has been widely used as a medicinal plant, especially in Asia. We typically use the pistil of the flower – going back to sixth-grade biology, the female reproductive part. The main chemical components of saffron are crocin (no, not the paracetamol brand), picrocrocin and safranal.

This precious spice effectively treats heart disease, high BP, stomach disorders, painful periods and learning and memory impairments. I have already pointed out how the stomach, circulatory system and mental health are affected in the winter. A pinch of saffron can be a very beneficial addition to your diet as you navigate these changes. Additionally, studies have indicated that saffron has anti-inflammatory (great for offsetting winter inflammation), anti-atherosclerotic (protects blood vessels), antigenotoxic (delays ageing) and cytotoxic (protects the stomach and joints) properties.

A few months ago, my husband went to Dubai and brought back some kick-ass quality saffron. That too at a good price since he knew a wholesale dealer. I kid you not, it has been a game changer for my kid's health. Nowadays I add four or five strands of saffron along with sugar to a glass of warm milk for his evening snack. I let the saffron soak in the milk for ten minutes before serving. The difference that this tiny habit has made to his health became obvious within just a few days.

With the reopening of schools, our kids have been re-exposed to school-grade germs and communicable illnesses. One kid in the class sneezes and the rest fall down like dominoes. There have been weeks on end when my two little ones shuttled viruses back and forth – one recovering only for the other to catch a viral and so on. My son was prone to chest congestion even after a case of simple sniffles, which meant only one thing: post-tussive vomiting, or puking because of coughing up so much mucus non-stop. It would take a long time for him to recover even after the viral had subsided and he would end up needing nebulization every so often.

Enter saffron in his evening milk. I first added it only because I wanted to use up the supply at home but the effect was as clear as day. My son's viral infections lasted for a shorter time. Upper respiratory tract infections did not trigger bronchitis and his seasonal allergies reduced significantly. Scientific evidence has confirmed the anti-cough effect of the stigmas and petals of the saffron plant – nature's cough syrup, if you must. The warming nature of the food improves immunity against respiratory infections. Saffron naturally has an anti-histaminic effect (nature's very own Cetirizine) that reduces sinus and lung secretions during infections. It has an expectorant effect too, i.e., it can help expel phlegm and reduce wheezing.

At this point I want to point out that unfortunately, there is no nutritional parameter used to determine the commercial quality of saffron (except moisture to prevent weight fraud). We know that quality depends on the source and imports from Iran and Afghanistan are at the top, with Super Negin saffron considered the world's best. However, Kashmiri saffron gives it a stiff competition when it comes to buyer loyalty.

There are few ways to assess whether the saffron you are buying is the real deal:

- **Soak the strands in water.** This will leech out the colour of the saffron. Real saffron will stay crimson red in a pool of yellow water while fake saffron will stain the water reddish with artificial dye.
- **Analyse its smell and taste.** Real saffron smells sweet and tastes bitter. If the fragrance or texture is off, chances are that it is fake. I once threw a clump of saffron into my biryani masala without mixing it well. By some stroke of luck, I was the one who got a mouthful of saffron's bitterness!

- **Opt for dark red saffron strands** and whenever you can, **avoid buying ground saffron**. It is easier to adulterate powder and the flavour in strands lasts longer.

For those who suffer from insomnia and other sleep-related problems, saffron has a relaxing and calming effect. Like a natural sleeping pill, it gently lulls the user into blissful sleep. Research shows that saffron increases glutamate and dopamine levels in the brain (Vata modulating effect). Glutamate is the chemical that accumulates in your brain when you have been engaged in rigorous mental activities like office work or studying. A midday nap goes a long way to relax you by eliminating glutamate from the brain during rest. The best way to consume this sleep-inducing spice is to mix a few strands into a glass of lukewarm milk. Milk contains the amino acid tryptophan, which is the raw material for the sleepy hormone melatonin, while saffron provides the sleepy chemical glutamate. Drink up and enjoy a good night's sleep provided by nature.

Saffron water is also helpful if you have PCOS or spotty periods. The chemical constituent anthocyanin in saffron reduces testosterone, normalizing the hormonal increase caused by PCOS to an extent. Spotty periods – in which you experience spotting for a couple of days before Aunt Flow comes to town – can be a pain. Quite literally and figuratively. Saffron also reduces the spasming of uterine vessels. This has a two-fold effect:

reduced period pain and easier blood flow. This next remedy is for my PCOS ladies.

Remember that saffron is a hot food. If you go by what the internet is telling you (I've seen websites recommend a dose of 30 mgs – anywhere between ten to fifteen strands – per day), you are in for a battlefield in your undies. The bleeding will be on an epic scale! Instead, have three or four strands per day – even five, depending on the potency of the saffron you are using. Soak them for fifteen minutes and consume the water in the morning. If you have regular but troublesome periods, start this process five or six days before your period is due to avoid spotting. As a bonus, you'll get relief from pesky PMS symptoms – moodiness, cramping, bloating, the works!

Saffron, packed with potent antioxidants, is also emerging as a top nutraceutical in brain health research. Studies suggest it may help protect brain cells after a stroke by reducing inflammation and oxidative damage, slow the growth of certain brain tumours by inhibiting cancer-cell proliferation, and improve memory and cognitive function in Alzheimer's disease by reducing amyloid-beta buildup and supporting neurotransmitter balance. A very striking and debilitating long-term effect of diabetes is nerve damage. This starts in the nerves that are farthest from the brain – those in your feet. Patients experiencing diabetic neuropathy (nerve illness) are tormented by the sensation of pins and needles. Saffron has shown promising results in reducing this nerve damage because of its antioxidant action.[41]

While I have harped on and on about saffron, I know full well that not everyone can afford to include it in their daily diet. Neither is it devoid of side effects. While researching saffron, I used to drink this amazing saffron milk tea (essentially normal chai with the spice added in towards the end of the brewing process). My periods did thank me for it but not so much my acne. My skin broke out like a teenage boy's, which brought me to the end of my honeymoon with saffron. Just like any other spice or herb, I realized I had to moderate my intake and not indulge in kesar chai so often.

Flaxseed – the most useful

Hate it or love it, flaxseed is here to stay. What started off as neglected cattle feed is now gaining popularity as a superfood that can nourish your hair and reduce cholesterol. It provides stability as well as flexibility to your cell membranes and stops the arteries of your heart from hardening. Softer arteries, softer hair and brainier children; this is the promise of flaxseed. One nutritionist will recommend that you chew and swallow it with water. Another will ask you to grind and sprinkle it over your morning muesli. Just like coconut oil, flaxseed is in a mercurial relationship with the public and media – love today, hate tomorrow. People just don't know when to stop with this wonderful seed.

Here is a fun tidbit: Flaxseed's scientific name is *Linum usitatissimum.* The second tongue-twister of a word means 'most useful'. And it lives up to the name!

Its fibres give us linen; we extract oil from the seed and make cakes to feed cattle as a byproduct. This in turn improves the quality of their milk. The active nutrient in flaxseed, lignan, has anti-inflammatory, antioxidant, anti-cancer, anti-bacterial, cholesterol-lowering and neuroprotective properties. Its consumption protects us from diabetes, Lupus, heart, kidney and bone disease. In women, it lowers the risk of hormone-dependent cancers and eases menopause symptoms.

A nutritionist advised one of my patients to consume ground flaxseed powder with water once a day during pregnancy. If you ask me, that sounds a bit like a TikTok challenge! The omega-3 content of this seed makes it fantastic for pregnant and breastfeeding mothers because it promotes brain development in the baby. However, flaxseed powder isn't very palatable – having to chug it daily is unsustainable. You don't have to torture yourself in the name of health. Instead of filling up your mouth with dry flaxseed powder and chasing it with a glass of water, try my mother-in-law's yummy ***flaxseed chutney recipe***:

Dry roast flaxseeds with whole Byadgi red chillis and garlic. Add salt and grind to a fine powder. Store this mixture in an airtight glass container and consume within two to three weeks. One tablespoon of dry flaxseed chutney with lunch is sufficient for the day. Just like dry idli-podi or gunpowder, you can relish your flaxseed chutney with dal, sabzi and ghee.

You can even add a tablespoon of ground flaxseeds to

your atta while kneading dough. It has a very subtle taste that will not interfere with the flavour of your meal. During pregnancy and after delivery, it is safe to consume one teaspoon of flaxseed chutney every day with lunch. A rich source of fatty acids, it keeps you full for longer and is excellent for your baby's brain development.

The first tenet of consuming flaxseed is to grind it. The nutrients pass untouched through your gut if the seed is consumed whole, so your body will not be able to reap its benefits. Another important issue to keep in mind is that the high omega-3 content in flaxseed powder makes it prone to oxidation. Once ground, consume it within two weeks and always keep it in an airtight container to prevent it from going rancid. Finally, limit your daily dose of flaxseed. It is human nature to go overboard when something comes with such a host of benefits but overconsumption will cause more harm than good. 15 g or one tablespoon of flaxseed powder a day is sufficient. An important side effect to bear in mind is that the lignan present in flaxseed mimics oestrogen (the female hormone). Overuse can affect one's ability to conceive and increase period flow.

Above and beyond the omega-3 call of duty, the hot nature of flaxseeds benefits our health in several ways.

1. **Mental health during winter:** In Ayurveda, flaxseed is given the special status of being a *Medhya*, or brain booster. The pro-inflammatory changes in our body during winter make us prone to feeling blue and can even trigger episodes of depression. Cortisol –

the stress hormone – is greatly reduced by flaxseed. Another blood marker, plasma fibrinogen, shows a slight increase in response to acute or chronic stress. Flax lignan regulates both these stress markers and stabilizes one's mood. Learn to bake flaxseed muffins, the ultimate comfort food.

2. **Bone health:** With menopause comes a dip in oestrogen, also known as our protective hormone. This hormone protects a woman from cardiovascular disease, osteoporosis and cognitive decline. Flaxseed has a weak oestrogen-mimicking action and consuming it daily after menopause protects against bone thinning. Flax lignans help keep the spine strong, and when taken with a doctor-prescribed low dose of oestrogen, they offer even better protection against post-menopausal bone loss.
3. **Better gut function:** A fantastic source of soluble fibre, flaxseed helps bulk up stool and prevent constipation – all too common in winter. The protein and fibre content also adds to your satiety, making you less likely to reach for another helping at lunchtime.
4. **Dealing with autoimmune disease:** Raynaud's phenomenon is a condition in which the blood vessels in one's fingers spasm due to stress or cold temperatures. The fingers turn pale and blue. Though the condition is not life threatening, it is extremely uncomfortable as the patient is not able to use their hands until the spasms subside and blood flow resumes. Flaxseeds have a high concentration of the

plant anti-inflammatory nutrient SDG, so a mere tablespoon of flaxseed daily can combat the agony of this condition.

Other Functional Seeds

There has been a very welcome surge in seed consumption because the media has hyped them up as 'nutraceuticals' – basically a fancy way to commercialize our staples. Nutrition plus pharmaceuticals equals nutraceuticals! Flaxseed was catapulted to stardom thanks to this movement. Pumpkin and sesame seeds followed suit. Let me give you a quick rundown of the health benefits of these hot-natured seeds. You'll have to wait until the cold foods chapter for the Kardashians' favourite, chia seeds.

Pumpkin seeds – tiny seeds, mighty deeds

1. **Protection from diabetes, high blood pressure and high cholesterol:** The fatty acid composition of pumpkin seeds makes them an excellent heart-healthy food. A great sugarless snack to munch on while you chit-chat with family on lazy evenings! Low in sodium and high in potassium, they protect against high BP. Their protein content is high – comparable to legumes – making them very satisfying. That means fewer cravings and binges.
2. **Food for racing thoughts:** A study assigned an antidepressant food score (AFS) of 47 per cent to pumpkin seeds. Feel like stress eating? Put pumpkin

seeds on the menu! Sleepless because you can't stop overthinking? Pumpkin seeds to the rescue with tryptophan, an amino acid that induces quality sleep. Anxious and irritable? Pumpkin seeds reduce jitteriness by bringing down glucose levels and increasing serotonin, your brain's happiness hormone.

3. **Men's health:** Every man will develop Benign Prostatic Hyperplasia (BPH) with age. The prostate gland (located at the base of the bladder) enlarges in size, compressing the urinary outflow tract over time. This results in poor urinary flow and frequent urination. Not dangerous, just a nuisance. Pumpkin seeds regulate male hormones and slow down this age-related prostate growth. Consuming them also improves erectile function and sperm health. Refer to Chapter 12 for directions for consuming pumpkin seeds for BPH.
4. **Worm expulsion:** Used in traditional medicine to expel intestinal worms, particularly in children. Try a simple blend of one teaspoon of raw pumpkin seeds mixed with honey on an empty stomach for a few days.

Sesame seeds – a powerhouse of minerals

Tahini has taken the food blogging world by storm. And for good reason! Its buttery, creamy taste makes it an out-of-the-world condiment, able to raise even the simplest recipes to divinity. It is derived from the humble sesame seed – and inherits its hot nature – whose benefits are too many to list. To name a few:

1. **Lactation food:** Tahini halva is a delicious comfort food that promotes postpartum recovery. It boosts milk production in new mothers and its calcium content ensures that mothers recover the calcium they secrete into their milk.
2. **Balancing your meal:** The humble hummus, though simple, is a delicacy you can't really go wrong with. Boiled chickpeas, garlic and tahini are ground to a fine paste that is usually devoured with a drizzle of olive oil and pita bread. Chickpeas are notorious for causing gas and have a cooling effect on the body. Tahini helps balance the nature of hummus, making its enjoyers less susceptible to the post-chickpea bloat.

Functional Vegetables

It's not just edible seeds that are being clubbed under the functional foods umbrella – the vegetables we ran away from as kids are also being given that label. Yes, they are functional and have always been. Their function is to fill our stomachs and keep us healthy. Alas, we feel the need to get permission from scientists before eating sabzi. Roti hasn't earned their stamp of approval just yet, since science still has a problem with gluten and carbs. I have faith, though. Just like a teenager eventually understands their parents were right all along, science too shall follow suit. It's just a matter of time.

Tuber vegetables are typically rich in phytonutrients such as betalains (beets), anthocyanins (purple yams), carotenoids (like beta-carotene in carrots), polyphenols and resistant starches. These compounds offer anti-inflammatory, antioxidant and neuroprotective benefits. Some tubers, like beet and radish, have mild diuretic properties, supporting kidney function and reducing water retention. This also helps check BP when it increases in winter because of blood redistribution. Tuber vegetables are generally easy to digest when cooked, offering warmth and nourishment. The resistant starch they contain feeds gut microbiota, promoting healthy digestion. However, when undercooked or eaten in excess, they may cause bloating in people with sluggish digestion or aggravated Kapha. The antioxidants and complex carbs in tubers support stable blood sugar, which is crucial for steady production of neurotransmitters like serotonin and dopamine. For example, the B-vitamins and tyrosine in sweet potatoes assist in dopamine synthesis, improving mood and cognitive function. Meanwhile the nitrates in beets enhance blood flow, including cerebral circulation, supporting mental clarity and focus.

One functional vegetable which has made waves in the food science community is beetroot. In the year 2014, beetroot was proven to be absolutely fabulous at regulating high BP.[42,43] But even more surprising was the effect it had on the inner lining of arteries, the endothelium. Endothelial dysfunction is the first step towards clogged arteries and heart attacks. The endothelium converts dietary nitrates into nitric oxide, one of the most important biological messengers in the body. It causes the muscles of the arteries to relax to allow increased blood flow. Beetroot stood out because it is an excellent source of nitrates.

Nitrate-rich foods enable muscles to extract more energy from the oxygen delivered by your blood. This finding, something not even conceived in physiology, was enough to make scientists question their own fundamentals. Nitrates not only deliver a higher quantity of blood to the muscles by dilating blood vessels but also enable tissues to extract more energy from the same quantity of blood and oxygen. One team of researchers gave trained divers 70 ml of nitrate-rich beetroot juice before a dynamic 75-metre swim underwater. After the dives, their blood oxygen level was higher compared to the placebo group.[44] This suggests that beetroot juice has an oxygen conserving effect.

Dietary nitrates also increase the capacity for ATP production in the mitochondria of muscles. ATP is basically the energy currency in your body – when you consume food, your mitochondria generate ATP that you use as energy. This increase in ATP production capacity after eating nitrate-rich foods occurs in the absence of any increase in the number of mitochondria. Research has shown that nitrates enhance mitochondrial coupling efficiency. In simple words, nitrates decrease energy 'wastage', effectively increasing the amount of ATP generated per unit of oxygen consumed.

Still sceptical about hot and cold nature of foods? The nitrate content in vegetables is higher in autumn than in spring, adding to the Vata-balancing property of these veggies.

Still confused whether you should increase oil intake in the winter? Sautéing vegetables in oil makes their nitrate content more available to you – a good 150 per cent increase in their bioavailable nitrate content as compared to raw vegetables.

Still torturing your taste buds by eating only boiled and steamed vegetables? Science gives you *ashirwaad* to stop! Boiling vegetables significantly lowers their nitrate content, quite literally sending the benefits you were looking for down the drain.

Traditionally, root vegetables are consumed more in the winter and this is a tradition I totally vouch for. The smell of gajar ka halwa wafting from the kitchen; beetroot palya and rotis for lunch; comforting aloo parathas for breakfast ... that is the winter we should be looking forward to.

A Quick Guide to Your Winter Diet

Hot or heating foods in Ayurveda

Fruits

- Dates
- Figs (dried)
- Pomegranates (ripe)
- Cherries
- Apples (slightly sour)

Vegetables

- Garlic
- Onions
- Leeks
- Radish
- Ginger (fresh or dried)
- Mustard greens

Grains and Legumes

- Wheat (especially in baked or cooked form)
- Chickpeas
- Lentils (mung, masoor and toor in cooked form)

Dairy

- Ghee (warming effect on digestion)
- Warm milk with spices (turmeric, ginger)
- Paneer (cooked in warming dishes)

Herbs and spices

- Black pepper
- Cinnamon
- Cloves
- Turmeric
- Ginger
- Mustard seeds
- Asafoetida

Beverages

- Ginger tea
- Spiced milk (turmeric, cinnamon, cardamom)
- Warm water with black pepper or cumin

Mechanisms of heating foods

1. **Stimulation of digestion:** Ushna (hot) foods enhance Agni (digestive fire), improving nutrient absorption and metabolism.
2. **Circulation and thermogenesis:** Spices like ginger and black pepper increase blood flow and internal heat, countering cold Vata tendencies.
3. **Vata pacification:** Warm, oily and cooked foods ground dry, light and cold Vata energies, reducing anxiety, lethargy and cold extremities.
4. **Immune support:** Many warming spices and herbs have antimicrobial and anti-inflammatory properties, enhancing resistance to winter infections.
5. **Mood and energy support:** By stimulating metabolism and circulation, these foods help maintain energy levels, warmth and emotional stability in the colder months.

Starting a winter diet

Principles

- Favour warm, cooked and slightly oily foods over raw, cold or dry foods.
- Include sweet, sour and salty tastes in moderation to balance Vata.

- Emphasize warming spices in cooking and beverages.
- Avoid excessive cold beverages, raw salads or overly astringent foods.
- Prioritize dense, grounding grains and legumes paired with warming herbs.

Recommended foods

- Warm porridge (wheat, barley, oats) with ghee and spices
- Soups and stews with root vegetables, lentils and mild spices
- Roasted nuts and seeds
- Warm milk with turmeric, cinnamon or ginger
- Cooked seasonal vegetables like carrot, beetroot and pumpkin

Dietary home remedies for cold Vata imbalance

1. **Ginger-honey tea:** Warm water with grated ginger and a teaspoon of honey supports digestion and circulation.
2. **Spiced milk:** Milk boiled with turmeric, cinnamon and cardamom promotes warmth and nourishes tissues.
3. **Warm cumin water:** Soak one teaspoon of cumin seeds in hot water, strain and drink to enhance digestion. A great remedy to get rid of bloating.
4. **Ghee-drizzled porridge:** Oats or wheat porridge with a teaspoon of ghee supports intestinal function and makes digestion easier.

5. **Roasted nuts and seeds:** Munch on nuts as they are a storehouse of excellent fats to nourish your hair, skin and nails. Lightly roasted almonds, walnuts and sesame seeds are great to snack on when curled up on your couch. As a bonus, say goodbye to winter blues with these brain foods.

9

YOUR BODY IN THE SUMMER

As the sun begins to shine for longer, the body gears up to go into reproduction and growth mode. The fat beneath the skin (the subcutaneous fat) automatically reduces irrespective of whether exercise was on the menu or not. Even in our weather-proof, air-conditioned homes, designed to shield us completely from seasonal changes, our bodies still follow nature's cues – packing on extra fat in winter to stay warm then trimming it down in summer to help with cooling. Researchers at Hokkaido University School of Medicine studied ten healthy males to investigate the influence of seasonal variations across five distinct seasons. They found that seasonal changes significantly impacted the natural physiological rhythms of the subjects. These included the timing of sleep onset, fluctuations in core body temperature throughout the day, average body temperature changes through the day and peak secretion of the circadian hormone melatonin. The subjects tended to retire to bed earliest during the summer months, followed by intermediate timings in spring and autumn, while winter saw the latest bedtime patterns. Wake-up times exhibited a parallel but more pronounced seasonality, with earlier awakening in summer.[45]

These observations testify to the correlation between human behaviour and seasonal changes. Our natural inclination towards early-to-bed, early-to-rise during summer reflects an adaptive response rooted in evolutionary history. Given early humans' reliance on natural light for daily activities such as hunting and agriculture, our biological clocks have evolved to optimize energy utilization from this primary light source.

Hotter weather in the summer also impacts sensory nerve responses. The skin's nerve receptors may become more sensitive to heat, leading to increased perception of warmth that may cause discomfort. In response to higher temperatures, nerve signals facilitate heat loss through increased blood flow to the skin. Nerves execute the body's thermostat mechanisms and signal the skin to sweat in order to cool it down.

The body's metabolic rate also reduces to control innate heat production. Our resting metabolic rate (RMR) is higher in the colder months. As we progress from winter to spring to summer, RMR wanes. The dip is quite significant – a decrease of about 20 per cent compared to winter. Summer also brings with it reduced appetite to lower heat production. In the case of seasonal switches in appetite, hot weather is the direct cause rather than changes in food intake.[46]

In nature, fat is used to protect animals from the biting cold. A bear enters winter hibernation all plump and emerges lean, as its body has used that excess fat to sustain itself. What a foolproof way to achieve the summer beach body! A study of female university students discovered somewhat similar patterns in human physiology. Subcutaneous fat increased in winter and decreased in summer, regardless of exercise. Upper body muscle mass also tends to drop in the summer due to reduced food intake, lowering resting metabolism and regulating body temperature. In contrast, lower limb muscle mass increased in the summer due to increased outdoor activity. While muscle changes are tied to diet and activity, fat gain appears to be seasonal.

Our skin is the next organ I want to explore. It is a living ecosystem, housing everything from microscopic mites to fungi to protective bacteria. A study of women aged eighteen to eighty in Shanghai found that, while visible ageing signs like wrinkles didn't change seasonally, skin functions did. In the summer, skin tone darkened and oil production and hydration increased, giving the subjects plumper skin. This effect wasn't down to the sudden appearance of extra oil glands, but increased activity by existing ones.[47]

Going a step further, not only do certain bodily diseases get aggravated seasonally but also our body's response to medication. The metabolism of fat (adipose) tissue is a great example of this. Adipose seasonality, as it is called medically, is a significant factor in obesity and metabolic disease. The efficacy of Thiazolidinediones (don't even try to pronounce it) – a commonly prescribed anti-diabetes medicine group – also varies by season. The responsiveness of the receptors it acts on changes throughout the year. This is a wake-up call for modern medicine practitioners: you need to introduce guidelines to adjust medication seasonally.

The Heat and Your Hormones

Summer is the season for making babies. The bodily changes that come with warmer weather tilt our hormone and immune systems in favour of reproduction. Shorter nights and longer sun exposure reduce melatonin and adrenocortical hormone secretion. In this state, the body ends up with lower overall inflammation and a calmer, more regulated immune state. A slightly suppressed or 'less vigilant' immune system makes it easier for the body to accept a fertilised egg which is, biologically speaking, half foreign. In winter, adrenocortical hormones run higher and the immune system is more reactive – great for fighting infections but not as ideal for implantation. In summer, the immune system naturally takes a step back, improving the uterus's receptivity by reducing inflammatory signals that might otherwise interfere with conception.

Melatonin is a key hormone tied to our daily and seasonal rhythms, regulated by the light-dark cycle. It helps restore the body and modulates immunity by shifting T helper cells towards Th-1 responses – essential for fighting infections. In contrast, excess Th-2 activity is linked to allergies. As the seasons shift, the extent of melatonin secretion changes. In summer, longer periods of daylight (photoperiod) and shorter periods of dark (scotoperiod) result in reduced melatonin production. Less melatonin means fewer Th-1 cells and more allergy-prone Th-2 cells, leading to those pesky summer allergy flare-ups. This is the main mechanism of seasonal allergies common in the spring season.

Prolactin is a hormone produced at night. Its most well-known function is milk production in lactating mothers but in males, prolactin tempers testosterone activity. This drives an urge to take care of the children one already has rather than reproduce. The longer winter nights offer more time to produce prolactin, while shorter summer nights mean less time to produce prolactin, a free reign for testosterone and an amped up sex drive. The shorter nights also hasten growth hormone production. Outdoor play during summer vacations combined with the God-gifted growth hormone surge at night is the best recipe for children's physical development.

Soil and the Season

We seem to have forgotten that the land we walk on and the air we breathe give life to the crops we grow. The seasons affect soil and produce – particularly fresh produce. There are two largely accepted models of seasonal food: global seasonality and local seasonality. Both describe food that is cultivated during the natural growing period for the region where it is produced. Neither require additional energy, reducing greenhouse gas emissions. But there is a key difference. Global seasonal food is not necessarily consumed in the same region and often goes into a box marked 'export', whereas local seasonal food is consumed regionally. This helps save our planet from the carbon footprint of storing and transporting food.

You might be surprised to learn that soil breathes, though not in the same way we do. The carbon stored in soil gets oxidized and released into the air as carbon dioxide. Later, carbon can return to the soil when plants and animals decompose. Here's the catch: as the year moves from February to August, the amount of organic matter and carbon in the soil drops. This goes hand in hand with a decline in soil microorganisms.

Microbial communities in soil and their enzyme activity – central to healthy ecosystems – are highly responsive to environmental shifts like temperature and rainfall. There's an intricate interplay between soil microbes, seasonal crop cycles and the animals (including us) that consume these crops. Soybeans, for instance, are planted in summer but bloom only in winter when daylight drops below twelve hours a day – a pattern seen in temperate regions of China. In another study focusing on the metabolism and absorption of soybeans in horses, researchers found that the byproduct of soy digestion – equol – was present in large quantities in the urine of female horses during the summer months but was minimal during the winter. This showed that the bacteria responsible for breaking down soy in the horse's digestive system are more active during the summer season. As the seasons shift, so does the soil's microbial activity. The soil itself changes, too. Its texture – or how it clumps together to form little lumps called aggregates – varies across the year. These shifts happen because of rising soil temperature and interactions between roots and microbes.

Think about how some fish swim alongside sharks, eating the dirt and parasites off their bodies. The fish get protection and the sharks get a free cleaning service. This is called symbiosis – a give-and-take between two living beings. Something similar happens underground as beneficial fungi form symbiotic relationships with plant roots, helping to bind the soil together like a hidden underground net. During the summer, when these fungi are most active and widely dispersed, the soil is more stable and less likely to be displaced by the wind or rain. This invisible canopy beneath the ground, formed by active roots and fungi, holds everything together.

In spring, winds carry away the top organic layer of soil. That's because the fields are left bare and the soil is unprotected by fungal growth in crop roots. A simple way to minimize this wastage of perfectly good soil is by growing so-called cover crops. You might remember studying about these in the fifth grade under crop rotation. Cover crops protect the soil while using different minerals from the primary crop. This allows the soil to rest, replenish and come back with a bang during sowing season. The need for fertilizer for the main crop also reduces, making the produce more organic.

Growing crops in unnatural habitats poses a big threat to soil quality and other environmental concerns. The cultivation of avocado in Portugal – a dry country – has placed a huge burden on a country already contending with water scarcity. Multiple batches are grown without giving the soil the opportunity to replenish its minerals and organic matter by using cover crops. It is unethical on so many levels to put our lands through this stress – and the people who live on it, too.

The *Khandaan* Effect

As urbanism progresses, community living regresses. However, there is a community in North America which has achieved the best of both worlds. The Hutterite community has embraced modern technology and medicine while maintaining a stable society rooted in communal living. You might notice some similarities to our big fat Indian khandaan.

Hutterites live in self-sufficient units they call colonies. Their three main meals are prepared and eaten in a colony dining room, using traditional recipes that have been preserved over time. The main source of variation in their diet is the seasonal availability of produce, which they primarily generate themselves. The summer season is for harvesting and preserving fresh produce and winters are for consuming the preserved produce. On this scale, the Hutterite clan – regardless of which colony they live in – pretty much eats in synchrony in their individual homes.

The researchers examined the gut bacteria of Hutterites across the seasons. The only difference in their diet was that fresh produce was consumed in summer and the produce they preserved by pickling or canning during winters. In accordance with other recent studies, over time the gut bacteria were stable across the population. The big surprise was that the bacteria got diverse over the summer and winter months across the community. These findings were unexpected because Hutterites share almost everything: their meals, environment, routines, even a relatively similar genetic background. Under such uniform conditions, scientists would expect their gut bacteria to look nearly identical throughout the year. Instead, the entire group showed coordinated seasonal shifts in microbial diversity, suggesting that external forces like temperature, daylight and humidity shape the gut far more strongly than individual habits. Thus, even in a tightly controlled, homogeneous community, nature still has the final say on how the microbiome behaves.

Weather impacts our gut bacteria more than we give it credit for – and not just in terms of seasonal eating habits. The bacteria respond to thermal (heat-related) and energy constraints. During dry periods, they specialize in breaking down starches found in underground plant parts (think tubers like potatoes).

During colder, drier seasons, bacterial genes involved in carbohydrate, protein and fat metabolism increase. This translates to increased fermentative activity and higher core body temperature to combat cold stress.

Just like our skin, teeth and hair are given love and care, our microbiome should also be treated and tended to. How, you ask? Bio-balance your diet based on the principles I've outlined and don't follow social media's recent addiction to whatever superfood they lay their hands on.

Starting Your Summer Diet

Histamines and sour foods

At this juncture, let me elaborate on histamines, the molecules I introduced in Chapter 5. They are present in immune cells and help our immune system identify and defend against threats. They are behind the watery eyes and nose, chest congestion, redness and flushing you might experience during a common cold or full-blown allergies. In essence, histamines are an integral part of our immune responses – even if those responses may be exaggerated sometimes, as in allergic reactions.

At times, the amount of histamine produced in or cleared from the body may fall out of balance. This lag can cause a condition known as histamine intolerance. It is more common than you would expect, though people are affected to different degrees. The human body is in a continuous state of mucus production. In fact, it produces a significant one litre of mucus daily. Sounds like a gooey mess, doesn't it? All this mucus goes on to protect your eyes from drying up and keep the respiratory and digestive passages moist and lubricated, shielding them from infections. The mucus layer is a rich source of the antibodies that defend your body from germs, and you have histamine-producing cells to thank for it.

Our gut produces an enzyme called diamine oxidase (DAO). In histamine-intolerant individuals this hormone is underproduced. Its crucial nature becomes clear when these individuals present with upper respiratory tract infections on consuming 'cold' foods that are often rich in histamines. Many patients have complained to me about developing throat pain or colds on eating sour foods like curd or pickles. The list of high-in-histamine foods is long: pickled fruits and vegetables, soy sauce, tomato ketchup, vinegar, curd and tomatoes. Add on fermented foods that are novel to Indians but prevalent in Southeast Asia such as kombucha, sauerkraut and kimchi.

Fermentation is a process which enhances digestibility by breaking down the proteins present in the parent food to simpler proteins and amines – histamine being the main one and tyramine its right-hand man. Together, this duo causes increased mucus production. DAO cannot deal with this amine-excess, adding to the mucus congestion from sour foods. The moral of the story is that if you are fighting a cold, steer clear of these foods. Your body is already producing too much mucus – don't add insult to injury and make the mucus stickier! I would even suggest avoiding dosa and idli during dinner in cold climates. I speak from experience, so pay attention, mommies. I've noticed that my Kapha-predominant kids have bouts of coughing when they consume dosas for dinner.

Both the digestive system and respiratory tract have receptors for histamine. Since histamine works locally, there is lots of crosstalk between the two systems via the histamine route. You don't have to snort a histamine-rich food to get mucus buildup in your respiratory tract. Mast cells in both the digestive and respiratory tracts release histamine in response to similar stimuli. Histamine released in one system can affect tissues and organs both distant and nearby. For example, a severe allergic reaction in the respiratory tract may lead to widespread histamine release and affect the gastrointestinal system. Medications that target histamine receptors, such as antihistamines like cetirizine or desloratadine, can also have widespread effects. An antihistamine taken for respiratory symptoms can influence digestive processes, leading to side effects like dry mouth and constipation.

Part of the reason that classic 'cold' fruits like banana and orange are labelled as such is their effect on histamine production. They boost histamine production, which then increases the body's tendency to produce mucus. That is why many suggest not eating these fruits after sunset. As the temperature dips in the evening, mucus production is revving up to protect the respiratory tract from the chill. If you are taking an antihistaminic like Allegra because of a runny nose, make sure to stay away from orange and lime – even if they are rich in vitamin C. The Allegra is blocking histamine's action to reduce mucus production even as the fruit increases histamine production. Kind of defeats the purpose of your cold medicine.

One last thing: customarily, whisky or brandy are suggested to combat the common cold. Alcohol may offer a false sense of warmth as it dilates the blood vessels in the skin, so the patient appears flush. But it is an offender when the patient is under the weather. Alcohol poses a triple threat to histamine-intolerant patients. It is rich in histamines, stops the histamine breakdown and triggers histamine release from our body cells.

Banana – the disgraced superfood

Today, banana carries the label 'fattening' and is universally feared by diabetics. Little do most people know that it was the first superfood ever!

If you are working out and want a snack that is portable and easy to eat, chuck the processed granola bar and opt for a handy banana instead. In addition to sustaining you through your workout due to its carbohydrate profile, banana's potassium content reduces water retention and tummy bloating. Sodium causes water retention and while 100 g of banana contains less than 1 mg of sodium, a 100 g granola bar is likely to have 300 mg of unnecessary sodium.

Aside from its brilliant potassium profile, the cooling properties of banana offer a fantastic menu of merits to benefit from.

1. An unripe/semi-ripe banana is loaded with resistant starch. This variety of starch is not digested in the small intestine and functions like fibre as it works its way to the large intestine. It's a great prebiotic, too.
2. Banana is nature's gut fixer. Constipated? Eat a banana. They contain soluble fibre known as pectin which eases constipation and normalizes motions. Diarrhoea? Eat a banana. The fibre profile of the banana absorbs water in the gut and reduces the quantity and frequency of motions. Heartburn because of acidity? Banana to the rescue. The mucus production kicked off by banana makes the mucus lining of the stomach thicker and more resilient to the onslaught of gastric juices and acid. Additionally, bananas contain protease inhibitors which help heal the damaged stomach lining and allay the discomfort of acidity and stomach ulcers.
3. Though bananas are not a rich source of calcium, their amazing potassium content promotes bone health. Potassium reduces calcium loss in urine – a common side effect of high-sodium diets (packaged food, I am looking at you!). So, every time you run after your child with a banana, tell them it will make their bones stronger.
4. The cold nature of bananas tempers excessive bleeding during periods. Consuming about a quarter

of a cooked banana flower mixed with a cup of curd is great for heavy flow. This combination increases progesterone levels and reduces bleeding caused due to hormonal imbalance.

5. The protein profile of banana, though not very rich, works as a great mood enhancer. One of the amino acids present in bananas, tryptophan, gets converted to serotonin – the happy hormone – when consumed.

It is a little unfortunate that I have to convince you to eat bananas (with, of course, a warning of when to avoid it as a cold food). This is a consequence of making tall 'superfood' claims. Let me burst your bubble: banana was the first ever superfood peddled to the public. This marketing campaign was launched way back during World War I – not by scientists or nutritionists but by the United Fruit Company.

United Fruit's primary business was controlling all aspects of cultivating and exporting tropical fruits – most notably bananas – from Latin American countries. The corporation was heavily criticized for exploiting and subjugating the local populations.[48] In the early twentieth century, United Fruit launched a campaign proclaiming bananas to be a superfood.[49] With the publication of studies citing the goodness of bananas, mainstream medicine adopted the fruit soon enough – for ailing patients, stronger bones, weaning babies. The handy fruit's peel became a cape in which it strut around as a superfood. Surrounded by this pro-banana messaging, ordinary homemakers latched onto the idea – a point of no return for any dietary craze.

Our devotion to and blind faith in these superfoods places them on a pedestal. Take blueberries, for example. A US government study once ranked them among the top antioxidant foods, leading to blueberries being promoted as a disease-fighting superfood. This ranking came from the USDA's ORAC (Oxygen Radical Absorbance Capacity) database, which measured the antioxidant capacity of foods in laboratory tests. However, these values did not necessarily reflect how antioxidants behave in the human body and the claims were largely overstated. Recognizing this, the USDA removed the database in 2012, cautioning that ORAC scores had been misused for marketing purposes and had limited relevance to real human health outcomes. Unfortunately, the new guidelines didn't have much of an effect on the popularity of blueberries. And that, my dear friends, is the power of promotion amongst the homemaker demographic.

Mango – king of the summer

Mango is the perfect summer food, replete with antioxidant goodness and digestive benefits. When it's hot, your mitochondria get stressed and produce harmful substances called reactive oxygen species (ROS). These ROS can harm the mitochondria, affecting their ability to produce energy and causing problems with your body's metabolism. Eating mangoes reduces the oxidative stress the summer heat imposes on your body by supplying natural antioxidants such as vitamin C, beta-carotene and polyphenols that neutralize free radicals and protect cells from heat-induced damage.

A very important tenet of eating mango is soaking the fruit in water for at least an hour before consumption. This reduces its phytic acid and tannin content. Once these anti-nutrients are out of the way, your digestive system can absorb micronutrients much better. Mangoes contain native digestive enzymes such as amylases (break down starch into sugars) and proteases (help digest proteins). Soaking at room temperature reactivates these enzymes, helping pre-digestion and reducing the glycaemic load to an extent. According to Ayurveda, mango is good for digestion due to its Deepan (appetizer), Pachan (digestion) and Pitta-balancing properties. It helps improve Agni, leading to a good appetite and enhanced metabolism.

Mangoes have other health benefits too, as follows:

1. **Diaphoresis:** During hot summers, our sweat glands become more active to cool down the body via sweat evaporation. Mango-based products induce a rise in body temperature, triggering sweating and alleviating heat stress. Mango's high water and electrolyte content replenishes fluids and minerals lost during sweating, especially in hot weather when fluid loss is significant.
2. **Gut function:** Mango is packed with dietary fibre, both soluble and insoluble. Soluble fibre soaks up water in your gut, forming a gel that softens stools

and helps you go to the bathroom. Insoluble fibre adds bulk to your stool, keeping it regular and preventing constipation. Mango also contains enzymes like amylase and lactase which aid digestion, as well as acids like citric, malic and tartaric that give it flavour, help with digestion and keep things moving smoothly in your intestines.

3. **Fluid balance:** Sweating dehydrates your body, concentrating the sodium levels in your blood. Mango is loaded with potassium, which regulates blood pressure and helps your kidneys flush out excess sodium and water.

As Cool as a Cabbage

Among vegetables, the cabbage and its relatives – the cruciferous family – are the prototypical cold foods. Move over orange juice! Cabbage is a superb source of vitamin C and its juice is more effective to prevent deficiency. Another good thing is that it isn't sold in Tetra Paks yet. Packing juice in that way reduces its vitamin-y goodness. I would suggest steering clear of any food which comes with a label announcing its health benefits. Real food does not talk.

The cooling nature of cabbage manifests in two primary ways: Pitta pacification (moderate consumption) and Vata disturbance (high consumption).

Pitta pacification

Eating cabbage helps cool down excess heat in the body, reduce inflammation and soothe digestion – all of which are common issues when your internal fire (Pitta) is high in the summer.

- **Hydrating and cooling effect**: Cruciferous vegetables contain plenty of water and potassium, which may mildly promote urine production. This balances out their hydrating action – the diuretic nature promotes loss of heat via increased urination. Since these vegetables are low in protein, they don't significantly increase the 'pull' of fluid into blood vessels (colloid osmotic pressure), preventing unwanted fluid shifts in the body. Cabbage's potassium, magnesium and hydration-supporting profile helps prevent summer dehydration-related symptoms like muscle cramps, burning urine and heat fatigue. Its alkaline effect calms the urinary tract – another area aggravated by Pitta.
- **Modulating mitochondrial function**: One key group of compounds in cruciferous vegetables are glucosinolates, which contain sulphur and break down into active substances like isothiocyanates when eaten. A well-known isothiocyanate called sulforaphane is found in the cabbage family. It improves mitochondrial function by activating the Nrf2 pathway, which helps protect cells from oxidative stress by boosting antioxidant proteins and detoxifying enzymes. This reduces damage to mitochondria caused by reactive oxygen species (ROS) – a significant contributor to ageing, brain diseases and metabolic disorders.

- **Gastric relief**: Cabbage juice is an excellent remedy for stomach ulcers. In fact, cabbage boasts a fantastic mineral and protein profile. I know it does not dress the part of a protein-rich food but just peel a layer away to discover its goodness.
- **Burning feet**: Cabbage is one of the few vegetables that contains vitamin B12, which helps keep your nervous system functioning smoothly and is often recommended for people with diabetes. High blood sugar can damage nerve endings over time, leading to tingling, burning or numbness in the toes and feet – a common 'hot' symptom experienced by long-standing diabetics before complete loss of sensation. Like other cruciferous vegetables, cabbage is rich in vitamins C, K and B6 and folate. These nutrients support nerve health, blood cell formation and overall metabolic function. Additionally, the bitter compounds in cabbage help improve glucose tolerance, which may further protect your nerves by reducing blood sugar spikes.
- **Relief from breast engorgement**: Cabbage leaves are traditionally used to relieve breast engorgement because they act as a natural cold compress, reducing localized heat, swelling and inflammation. Modern evidence suggests that cabbage leaves help decrease tissue congestion and improve lymphatic drainage – an excellent example of their Pitta-pacifying, cooling and soothing properties. Refer to Chapter 13 for instructions on how to use cabbage leaves in this way.

- **Anti-inflammatory action and skin relief**: Cabbage contains anthocyanins, sulforaphane and high vitamin C, which collectively reduce inflammatory markers. This helps calm acne flare-ups, redness and irritation – all of which Ayurveda associates with aggravated Pitta. Its cooling water content makes it especially beneficial during summer, when there is a spike in skin issues due to the heat.

Vata disturbance

Eating too much cabbage – especially raw or in the cold season – can cause gas, bloating, sluggish digestion and even aggravate joint stiffness or arthritis. This is a result of its heavy and cold qualities that imbalance the airy, mobile nature of Vata in the body.

From an Ayurvedic perspective, cabbage and its family members are gas-formers. The paratha-*wala* cauliflower, beautiful broccoli and newly popular kale are all cousins. That is, they increase Vata dosha in the body, in large part due to a component called raffinose. Raffinose is a carbohydrate that, when consumed, passes through the stomach and small intestine undigested. Upon reaching the large intestine, it is fermented by bacteria. Gases such as carbon dioxide and methane are byproducts of this process. These can cause bloating, flatulence and discomfort, leading to the characteristic gassiness associated with the cabbage family.

Breastfeeding mothers should steer clear of the cabbage family. Raffinose is passed on via breastmilk. It accumulates and ferments in the baby's large intestine and can make them gassy or colicky.

A rheumatologist's nemesis

Have you heard of palindromic arthritis? This condition shows up as recurrent episodes of joint inflammation that come and go unpredictably. Episodes typically last between a few days to a week and affect one or multiple joints, causing pain, swelling and stiffness.

A palindrome is a word or phrase that reads the same forwards and backwards. For instance, the word Malayalam. This kind of arthritis is called palindromic because the joints are the same before and after an attack. Theoretically, such inflammation should cause some residual damage to the joint. However, remarkably, there is no lasting joint damage. Between episodes, symptoms resolve completely and the joints return to normal.

A thirty-four-year-old male patient once presented to a colleague of mine with palindromic arthritis. He reported that his joints had a tendency to swell up every single time he ate cauliflower. After two days, the swelling and pain would subside as if nothing had happened. He insisted that avoiding cauliflower was the only remedy to his condition.

Palindromic arthritis is a couple of steps away from rheumatoid arthritis. Cabbage is not particularly rich in protein compared to other food sources but it *does* contain an important amino acid, arginine. It also contains glucosinolates that can be converted into isothiocyanates like sulforaphane. Sulforaphane blocks an enzyme called arginase that is responsible for breaking down arginine. When this happens, the body retains more arginine.

Arginine can be turned into another substance called citrulline through a process called citrullination. This activity is normal and helps control genes or remove dying cells. But in people with rheumatoid or palindromic arthritis, citrullination goes overboard. The immune system starts seeing citrullinated proteins as enemies and produces special antibodies called Anti-CCP which attack the joints and cause pain, swelling and long-term damage.

Here's where the cabbage family acts as a double-edged sword. Patients with rheumatoid or palindromic arthritis often have a tendency to build up too much arginine. Vegetables like cabbage not only supply more arginine but their sulforaphane content also stops the body from clearing the excess. Too much citrullination creates new, altered proteins - neoantigens - that the immune system mistakes for intruders. For someone with an already hyperactive and sensitive immune system, this exacerbates joint inflammation. Essentially, in autoimmune arthritis, citrullination acts like a faulty alarm system that keeps ringing for no real reason - and cruciferous vegetables might unintentionally push the button.

These changes point to an increase in Vata - a new system of communication is formed through citrullination of the excess arginine present in the cabbage. The command of making aberrant changes to proteins after production is what is meant by Vata dosha increase.

Cabbage family meets the thyroid gland

Every cell requires the thyroid hormone for smooth functioning, from your brain cells to your uterus lining. The thyroid helps maintain body temperature, reproductive health, growth and optimal metabolism in the body (too much or too little are medical conditions that demand prompt and often continual attention). Brain growth and bone maturation in children both heavily depend on this gland's functioning. In case of a growth spurt or pregnancy, the demand for the hormone increases.

Members of the cabbage family reduce production of the thyroid hormone. The cold-causing nature of the cabbage plant opposes the thyroid hormone's function of keeping the body warm and metabolism high enough to maintain core temperature. A by-product of cabbage digestion is an anti metabolite compound known as thiocyanate. It stops the uptake of iodine to the thyroid gland, resulting in hypothyroidism. Patients suffering from hypothyroidism are advised to eat less cabbage because of this side effect.

It may seem like I would recommend avoiding cabbage if you are trying to conceive but that couldn't be further from the truth. Cabbage is totally fine to eat if you're planning a baby or have already conceived provided you don't have hypothyroidism. In fact, its high folic acid content is a boon for expecting moms. Rich in fibre, cabbage can also regulate sugar levels, making PCOS more manageable for women wishing to conceive.

Sauerkraut – a truly functional food

Sauerkraut is fermented cabbage. It is abundant in prebiotic – the fibre that feeds our gut bacteria and keeps them happy. It is also a probiotic because the fermentation process increases its helpful bacterial content. The gas production caused by eating raw cabbage is tempered through cooking and fermentation, as its carbohydrate structure is altered. This enables a whole host of benefits.

Allopathy often fails to recognize how the action of heat and salt can cause physical changes in our food. Fermentation in brine adds to the beneficial properties of cabbage and reduces Vata dosha. It promotes the release of gastric juices and smooth movement of food down the digestive tract. The acid component – lactic acid – in sauerkraut counteracts the growth of bad bacteria in your gut. A word of caution: if you have more bacteria in your small intestine than your large intestine (a condition called small intestinal bacterial overgrowth), you are likely to be bothered by any preparation of cabbage. Digestion of cabbage fibre by the small intestinal bacteria will produce more gas, resulting in a bloated belly.

Sauerkraut is high in vitamins C and K. The nutrient profile of cabbage also ensures that calcium is deposited in the bones, making them stronger. On the other hand, it removes calcification from your arterial walls, making them more elastic and decreasing blockages. The S-methyl-methionine component of cabbage helps heal ulcers and inflammation throughout the gut. The close-to-endless list of functions of sauerkraut make it the ideal functional food. If you are sceptical about its acidic taste, don't worry – it's safe to consume. But if your stomach is sensitive, steamed cabbage is a great alternative.

10

WHEN YOUR INSIDES HEAT UP: COOLING FUNCTIONAL FOODS

The long, sun-baked days of summer bring with them a natural increase in body temperature and perspiration. Eating cooling, hydrating foods that refresh and regulate the body is essential during this season. Certain health conditions can further elevate internal Pitta, causing inflammation, acne due to gastric issues, urinary tract or yeast infections. By choosing foods that calm internal heat and support gentle cooling, we can address heat imbalances – both seasonal and internal. This keeps our bodies comfortable, balanced and resilient throughout the hot months.

Barley – the Functional Grain

In Ayurveda, barley is called *yavam*. Charaka recognized it as the most effective among foods that promote healthy bowel movements, known as *Purishajanaka*. During my research, barley was the goose that laid the golden egg. The discovery that its cooling nature can help cool a woman's nethers was quite a surprise! If you are a man, you will not understand the agony of a urinary tract infection (UTI) or the unbearable itchiness of a yeast infection. But for the women reading, barley water is an awesome fix for UTIs and recurrent vaginal infections.

Yeast infections

Vaginal candidiasis, commonly known as a yeast infection, is a condition characterized by the overgrowth of the fungus Candida in the vaginal area. This leads to symptoms such as itching, burning and curdy white discharge. Yeast infections are more commonly seen in diabetics and can often recur despite treatment.

Interestingly, Ayurveda classifies vaginal candidiasis as a Kapha disorder. This aligns with the modern scientific understanding of the condition. Kapha is characterized by qualities such as heaviness, moistness and sweetness. I explained the mechanism of Kapha predominance in Chapter 2. During yeast infections we see a very similar mechanism of ECM overproduction. However, the overproduction in this case is by the fungus itself, using our body's resources.

Imagine your body as a bustling city with different types of microorganisms living together in harmony. Among these is a fungus called Candida, naturally present in small amounts without causing any trouble. However, sometimes Candida can grow out of control, leading to infections that are most common in warm, moist areas like the mouth, gut and vagina.

The Candida yeast cells adhere to vaginal surfaces and each other, multiplying and forming filamentous structures known as hyphae and pseudohyphae. These fungal structures accumulate a protective ECM that allows them to evade the host's immune response and antifungal treatments. This process, known as biofilm formation, is a hallmark of Candida infections. For candida's success as a pathogen, this biofilm is more like a bio-fortress! A living evolving fortress that lets it thrive despite the host's defences.

Moreover, the availability of glucose, often associated with sweet and heavy foods, enhances the virulence of this fungus. When Candida is under control in our body, it is present in budding form. But when it becomes the infective invader, it unleashes its branching form. Glucose has been shown to induce this branching form, promoting its growth and persistence. Dietary factors significantly contribute to the spread and severity of yeast infections, making it important to check the patient for diabetes and high sugar. Immune cells like macrophages also rely on glucose to survive and fight the fungus. Exploiting this vulnerability, Candida lays siege on the local immune cells by exhausting the accessible glucose.

Thankfully, our immune cells aren't a bunch of bozos. They employ a similar tactic, nutritional immunity, whereby the host's immune system attempts to withhold essential nutrients from the invading pathogen. This innate defence mechanism aims to limit the availability of nutrients that are necessary for the pathogen's survival, restricting its growth within the host. Basically, our body witnesses a starvation tug-of-war between our immune cells and the fungus. Both are trying to overpower the other by cutting off their food supply. A brilliant military tactic!

Vaginal good bacteria (Lactobacillus species) help maintain a healthy balance in the vaginal environment by producing lactic acid. This keeps the pH level acidic, preventing harmful bacteria and yeast from overgrowing and causing infections. These beneficial bacteria also produce substances that help protect against infections and support overall vaginal health. Several studies have suggested that beta-glucan, a soluble fibre found in barley, has a positive effect on vaginal health by modulating the composition and function of bacteria. Here's how barley – more specifically, beta-glucan – can save the day when things get itchy down there:

- Beta-glucan acts as a prebiotic, meaning it serves as food for beneficial bacteria in the vagina. This fermentation process produces SCFAs which help maintain an acidic pH that is inhospitable for pathogenic microbes.
- Beta-glucan promotes the recruitment and activation of immune cells in the vaginal mucosa to defend against pathogens.
- Chronic inflammation in the vaginal mucosa is associated with conditions like bacterial vaginosis and vulvovaginal candidiasis. Beta-glucan has been shown

to snub the inflammation by suppressing the pro-inflammatory cytokines and promoting the release of anti-inflammatory mediators.

- Beta-glucan strengthens the vaginal cell barrier by promoting cell multiplication, enhancing cell to cell integrity and increasing mucin production. This enhanced barrier function prevents the entry of microbes into the vaginal tissue. You can see evidence of barley's sweet and nourishing nature as it supports cell growth and tissue structure solidity.
- While beta-glucan does not possess direct antimicrobial properties, its fermentation products do.

Barley water is a time-honoured beverage in both Ayurveda and Unani. Barley possesses cooling properties that have been recognized for centuries – among them, its diuretic effect. Diuresis is the increased production of urine by the kidneys, leading to more frequent urination. This helps remove excess water and waste products from the body, promoting hydration and electrolyte balance.

How to make barley water: Rinse one cup of pearl barley, then soak it in four cups of water overnight. Bring the mixture to a boil in the morning and simmer for twenty to thirty minutes, until the barley is soft. Strain the barley water and allow it to cool before serving. Drink one or two glasses per day.

Urinary tract infections – water on fire

UTIs are among the most common bacterial infections. With antibiotic resistance on the rise, UTI management needs to turn to natural cures and home remedies. Not to mention that antibiotics, even when effective, disrupt the body's natural good bacteria. If you have a UTI and take an antibiotic, it not only targets the bladder bacteria but also bacteria in the gut and vagina (and mouth, nose and skin). It is quite common for women to notice white discharge after a course of antibiotics because their vaginal good bacteria have been disrupted.

Once again, turn to barley water – a possible be-all and end-all of your lady issues. White discharge? Check! Itchy vulva? Check! Burning urine? Check!

For an infection to take place, bacteria or fungus have to stick to the cells – a process called bacterial or fungal adhesion. What beta-glucan does is prevent the first step itself. There's no need to kill the bacteria because, faced with a non-stick Teflon coating, they simply get flushed out with urine. Beta-glucan also interacts with cell receptors and recruits immune cells.

The diuretic effect of barley also provides added UTI protection. Increased urine production and flow ensures that the bacteria are flushed out. This is an example of the 'drying' nature of barley. However, the beauty of this natural cure is that although it is drying, it does not cause constipation. In fact, the fibre content of barley absorbs water from the intestine and bulks up stool, making your bowel movements as smooth as it gets. In South India, barley water is given to those experiencing diarrhoea to hydrate the patient and reduce stool volume.

Man, nature has really got our back!

Barley and barely hanging in there

Talbina is a traditional Islamic remedy food prepared from barley. Aisha, wife of the Prophet Muhammad, peace be upon him, reported that he would recommend talbina whenever someone in his household fell ill. Customarily, it was made for grieving relatives during funerals. If you are faced with a tough situation in life or your mood is down in the dumps, make sure to try this soothing anti-depressant porridge.

The comforting porridge is cooling, grounding and easily digestible. Depression is often associated with Vata imbalance (dry, light, cold qualities) and at times with Pitta aggravation (heat, irritability). From a scientific perspective, the link between Vata disturbance and depression can be understood as imbalances in neurotransmitters such as serotonin and dopamine which govern mood and emotional stability. The cool and dry qualities of talbina help pacify aggravated Pitta and stabilize Vata, nourishing the nervous system to create a sense of mental calm.

How to make talbina: If using whole barley grains, rinse thoroughly and soak in water overnight to soften them. The soaked grains are then ground into a coarse or fine flour. Combine the barley flour with water or milk in a saucepan and bring the mixture to a gentle boil over medium heat, stirring continually to prevent lumps from forming. Once the porridge comes to a boil, reduce the heat to low and allow it to simmer for fifteen to twenty minutes, or until it reaches the desired consistency. Sweeten with honey as per your taste, along with cinnamon or cardamom powder for added flavour. Garnish with chopped nuts and dates before serving.

Dysbiosis, or imbalance in the gut microbiota, has been observed in patients with depression. This manifests as reduced levels of beneficial bacteria and overgrowth of harmful bacteria. Gut bacteria play a crucial role in regulating mood, behaviour and brain function through the gut-brain axis. Disruptions in the gut microbiome can contribute to neuroinflammation and neurotransmitter imbalances that are implicated in the pathophysiology of depression.

Depression has also been associated with increased gut permeability, also known as leaky gut syndrome. The lining of the intestines becomes more porous, allowing substances such as toxins, undigested food particles and bacteria to leak into the bloodstream. Chronic stress – a common component of depression – can aggravate gut permeability by disrupting the integrity of the intestinal barrier. Increased gut permeability is linked to inflammation and immune dysregulation, which can worsen depression.

Barley's potential modulation of anxiety and depression is achieved through several mechanisms.

1. **Gut microbiota modulation:** Barley promotes the growth of beneficial gut bacteria, which produce neurotransmitters such as serotonin and GABA that are involved in mood regulation.
2. **Stabilizing blood sugar levels:** Barley's low glycaemic index helps maintain stable blood sugar levels, preventing mood swings and anxiety associated with fluctuating glucose levels.
3. **Anti-inflammatory effect:** Barley's antioxidant and fibre content help reduce inflammation and oxidative stress, which are implicated in the development of mood disorders such as depression and anxiety.
4. **Rich in minerals:** Barley is a great source of manganese and selenium. Selenium helps protect nerve cells from damage caused by inflammation and oxidative stress. One of the key enzymes that selenium helps activate is glutathione peroxidase, which is critical for the metabolism of neurotransmitters like dopamine and serotonin. These are the happiness molecules in the brain that regulate our mood.

Other applications of barley

Here is a blitzkrieg list of barley's applications without turning this book into its biography:

1. **Diabetes:** Improves insulin resistance. Particularly useful if your post-food sugar is high. Can consume as barley water, porridge or khichdi.
2. **Heart disease:** Reduces fluid overload due to heart failure, reduces cardiometabolic risk and reverses the

damage caused by heart attacks. Patients experiencing these conditions should make barley a staple in their diet.

3. **High cholesterol:** Helps manage the body's lipid levels by increasing excretion and reducing (though not stopping) cholesterol production. Again, a win-win for heart disease.
4. **Blood pressure:** A very rich source of potassium and has a sodium-excreting effect. This makes it a good choice of grain for those with high BP.
5. **Stomach ulcers:** Fermented barley extract, rich in beta-glucan, protects the stomach from injury by reducing oxidative stress and inflammation. It lowers levels of malondialdehyde and enhances antioxidant defences. The extract's effects are comparable to omeprazole, a very effective antacid.
6. **Fatty liver:** Sprouted barley works great for reversing fatty liver.
7. **Chronic kidney disease:** Barley beta-glucans promote a healthier gut microbiota by decreasing blood levels of p-cresyl sulphate toxin and increasing production of fatty acids in the colon. This can lower the risk of uremic toxin build-up and circulatory issues in chronic kidney disease. For stage-3 chronic kidney disease patients, barley consumption significantly improves nutritional status and renal function.
8. **Post-Covid fatigue:** A study of Covid patients in Iran found that both low oxygen levels and fatigue improved on consuming barley water.[50] The flavone

compounds it contains improve oxygen supply to tissues – another example of Pitta pacification!

One of my lovely neighbours, Vedha aunty, told me that pregnant women are given barley water in Tamil Nadu to soothe swollen feet. Barley water is safe to consume daily during pregnancy. Eating barley a few times a week in the form of khichdi or porridge may help keep diabetes and high BP at bay during pregnancy. It also effectively reduces nausea, constipation, heartburn and of course, water retention.

A simple indication that you are consuming too much barley is sinus irritation and dry nasal surfaces. This is owed to its drying effect on the nose and sinuses. Avoid barley if you are sensitive to gluten.

Gooey Goodness: Sabja and Chia Seeds

Sabja or basil seeds are small black seeds obtained from the sweet basil plant (*Ocimum basilicum*). When soaked in water they expand and develop a gel-like coating, akin to chia seeds. Packed with fibre, vitamins and minerals, they are believed to possess cooling properties, making them a favoured ingredient in classic Indian summer refreshments such as falooda and sharbat.

Chia seeds (*Salvia hispanica*) originated in North and Central America and belong to the mint family. They were a vital part of the Aztec diet before European colonization. While chia is an awesome food, I'm a wee bit prejudiced against it because the mother of consumerism Kim Kardashian has become its self-appointed brand ambassador (colonial mindset much?). Moreover, the seed is not indigenous to India. Putting my biases aside, let's explore the greatness of sabja and chia.

The mucilage content of chia and sabja seeds offers a multitude of benefits for overall health and well-being. If you soak sabja or chia seeds in water, you will see how they absorb the liquid and swell up. The gel-like substance produced is alkaline and neutralizes excess stomach acid. In the month of Ramadan, Roohafza is served with soaked sabja during Iftar because of the seed's ability to alleviate thirst and acidity following the day-long fast.

Scientific studies show that mucilage polysaccharides like arabinoxylans and xyloglucans support the ECM and boost mitochondrial function, enhancing energy production and improving Pitta dosha. The water-loving mucilage hydrates and lubricates the ECM, safeguarding tissues against dryness and stiffness. This is the mechanism by which it improves Vata dosha as per Ayurveda. Also, mucilage forms a protective barrier within the digestive tract, shielding the intestinal lining from damage and inflammation, thus preserving intestinal cells. It maintains the structural integrity of connective tissues by supporting ECM stability, which prevents tissue degradation and fosters overall tissue health and function. It influences cell–ECM interactions, crucial for tissue repair and regeneration. In essence, the mucilage content in chia and sabja seeds offers a holistic boost to ECM health.

Oh and, by the way, drinks that contain sabja can tone down the burning sensation experienced during UTIs. You are welcome.

Coriander Seed – the Cool Spice

Coriander seeds (*Coriandrum sativum*) have been widely valued in traditional medicine and are gradually capturing modern scientific interest. They are rich in antioxidants such as quercetin, linalool and terpenoids which neutralize free radicals within mitochondria. Quercetin is also known to support mitochondrial biogenesis and energy regulation.

Traditionally used in digestive tonics, coriander seeds are considered both carminative and stomachic. Rather than aggressively stimulating stomach acid, coriander appears to have a modulatory effect. Studies show that coriander extract may reduce gastric ulcers and support mucosal defense, especially under stress conditions like alcohol consumption or excess painkiller use. This effect could be because it reduces irritation and shields the body like an antioxidant. Meanwhile it contains oils such as linalool that gently slow the stomach's acid production. The result is well-balanced acid secretion – sufficient for digestion but protective against excess acidity.

Blood pH is tightly regulated between 7.35 and 7.45 – a balance that coriander seeds may support indirectly. They are believed to have a mild alkalizing effect on urine and can assist acid-base homeostasis by promoting kidney function and reducing systemic oxidative stress. These actions help the body buffer metabolic acids more efficiently.

Natural Elixir: Tender Coconut Water

Tender coconut water, the clear fluid found inside young green coconuts, is revered in traditional medicine systems like Ayurveda for its cooling, hydrating and soothing properties. Rich in electrolytes, sugars, amino acids, vitamins and phytohormones, it is nature's perfect drink. Its multidimensional benefits extend to dosha balance, cellular metabolism, nervous system regulation, endocrine function and internal tissue protection.

Ayurvedic practitioners use tender coconut water for the cooling (*Sheetala*), unctuous (*Snigdha*) and sweet (Madhura) properties that make it a natural Pitta pacifier. It is especially beneficial during hot seasons or inflammatory conditions, alleviating symptoms like acidity, burning sensations, skin irritation and excessive thirst. Coconut water is best consumed fresh in the morning or midday on an empty stomach. Avoid it in cold weather or at night and use cautiously when experiencing Kapha conditions like sluggish digestion, sinusitis or diarrhoea. Always give preference to fresh over bottled coconut water.

Biomedically, coconut water supports mitochondrial function by supplying electrolytes (magnesium, potassium), glucose and antioxidants like ascorbic acid which help boost ATP production and reduce oxidative stress. The beverage helps reduce overactivity in the SNS due to heat or stress by quickly restoring electrolyte balance and supporting GABA function through its magnesium content. This makes it useful for calming nervous tension, palpitations and heat-induced irritability.

To the thyroid, coconut water offers trace minerals like selenium and zinc that support enzyme function. Its cooling nature can help manage Pitta-type hyperthyroidism by reducing heat and inflammation without overstimulating thyroid activity.

Though direct studies are limited, its hydrating and antioxidant-rich profile suggests benefits for serous membranes (pericardium, pleura, peritoneum). It helps reduce oxidative damage, prevent fluid imbalance and supports mesothelial health, aligning with the Ayurvedic concept of nourishing internal membranes.

Bhindi – the Mucilage Mistress

Bhindi or okra, celebrated for its therapeutic mucilage, holds a special place in both culinary and healing traditions. Rich in fibre, folate, vitamins C and K and minerals like magnesium, bhindi also contains mucilage – just like sabja and chia – that offers a multitude of health benefits, especially for the gut, metabolism and blood sugar regulation. When bhindi is sliced, this mucilage is what creates that characteristic slippery texture.

Mucilage is a prebiotic, supporting the growth of beneficial gut bacteria and regular bowel movements. Here is a shocker: consuming probiotics in drink or pill form isn't as beneficial as we have been led to believe. The resident bacteria in your gut put up a fight against the newcomers and eliminate them in a day or two. A more effective alternative to nourish our gut microbiome is soluble fibre. It bulks up in the gut and cements the mucosal lining of the intestines by lodging itself in the spaces between cells. This has a cooling effect on the mucosa and feeds your beloved bacteria. If your gut bacteria aren't fed, they go into a famine frenzy and start eating up the intestinal lining. Enter bhindi, with its sticky soluble fibre – mucilage.

In addition to feeding your bacteria, mucilage slows down carbohydrate digestion and absorption, reducing blood glucose spikes. It also binds bile acids in the gut and aids in cholesterol excretion, supporting heart health. The mucilage and phenolic content in bhindi may help control intestinal and metabolic inflammation. Thus bhindi is more than just a culinary staple – it's a functional food that offers metabolic, digestive and anti-inflammatory benefits.

Here's a concise guide to how cooking alters bhindi's properties to help you maximize its value in Pitta-pacifying, gut-soothing and glucose-regulating dietary strategies.

- **Dry sautéing** (e.g., bhindi fry): Reduces mucilage significantly due to dehydration, making it less slimy and more palatable.

- **Steaming or boiling**: Retains more mucilage, especially if cooked gently, preserving gut-soothing and metabolic benefits.
- **Cooking with acidic ingredients** like tomatoes or lemon can reduce slime by breaking down mucilage structure. For those with Kapha predominance, this cooking method mitigates the cooling effect of bhindi.
- **Deep-frying** denatures the mucilage and reduces its therapeutic value. Again, a safe way to eat bhindi for Kapha individuals.

To retain mucilage for health benefits, gentle cooking or raw-soaked preparations are preferred.

Bhindi (okra) chutney

This traditional South Indian-style chutney preserves some mucilage and combines the digestive and metabolic benefits of bhindi with gut-friendly spices.

Ingredients:

Fresh tender bhindi – 10–12, grated coconut – 2 tbsp, tamarind pulp – 1 tsp, green chili – 1 (optional), cumin seeds – 1/2 tsp

Directions:

Lightly sauté bhindi in ghee or oil until slightly softened but not browned. Cool and blend with coconut, tamarind, green chili, cumin and salt. Temper mustard seeds and curry leaves in oil, then add to the chutney. Serve fresh with rice or dosa.

This method preserves part of the mucilage while still making it palatable, combining soothing and digestive actions.

Bhindi water

Bhindi water is made by soaking sliced bhindi in water overnight. This method draws out the vegetable's mucilage and water-soluble antioxidants.

Upon consumption, bhindi water forms a viscous gel in the stomach that slows glucose absorption, supporting insulin sensitivity. This gel coats the gut, soothing acid reflux, ulcers and gastritis. It also improves bowel regularity and reduces irritation in the colon, relieving IBS and constipation. Those suffering from anal fissures stand to benefit from bhindi water as it hydrates and bulks up stools, making them much easier to pass. Its cooling, demulcent nature helps address internal heat and inflammation, curbing inflammatory acne.

Pitta-Pacifying Foods

Cooling foods help pacify aggravation of the Pitta dosha. Our bio-energies require modulation, not blind suppression. Your body signals ongoing disruption to Pitta in the form of symptoms which scream hot, hot, HOT! Some common symptoms include:

1. **Acid reflux**: Excessive acidity in the stomach leading to discomfort and a burning sensation in the chest.

2. **Ulcers**: Sores in the stomach lining or intestines causing pain and discomfort.
3. **Gastritis**: Inflammation of the stomach lining resulting in nausea, vomiting and belly ache.
4. **IBS**: Functional gastrointestinal disorder causing abdominal pain, bloating and altered bowel habits.
5. **Skin symptoms** like rashes, rosacea and acne.
6. **Hypertension**: High BP, often associated with stress and emotional factors.
7. **Excessive sweating** due to hyperactivity of the sweat glands.
8. **Migraines**: Recurring headaches often accompanied by nausea, sensitivity to light and sound and visual disturbances.
9. **Hyperthyroidism**: Overactive thyroid gland producing excessive thyroid hormones, leading to symptoms such as weight loss, rapid heartbeat and heat intolerance.

Pitta's tendency towards symptoms that feel 'hot' shows up at the cellular level, too. External temperature directly affects mitochondrial function. Excessive heat can cause mitochondrial overactivation, leading to the generation of more ROS, which damage cells. High temperatures can also impair mitochondrial enzymes and transport proteins, disrupting the electron transport chain.

Summer aggravates Pitta dosha. To restore balance, Ayurveda recommends foods that are cooling, hydrating and soothing. The three tastes most effective in pacifying Pitta are:

1. Madhura (sweet) – cooling and nourishing; found in milk, rice, ghee, dates, coconut water and sweet fruits like mango.
2. *Tikta* (bitter) – detoxifying and cooling; found in bitter gourd, neem, spinach and coriander.
3. *Kashaya* (astringent) – cooling and drying; found in pomegranate, green tea, okra and legumes.

In contrast, sour (Amla), salty (*Lavana*) and pungent (Katu) tastes aggravate Pitta by increasing heat, acidity and internal pressure. These are best avoided during summer.

A Quick Guide to Your Summer Diet

Cold or cooling foods in Ayurveda

Fruits

- Watermelon
- Pomegranate
- Coconut
- Grapes
- Apples (sweet)
- Pears
- Mango (ripe)
- Cherries
- Figs

Vegetables

- Cucumber
- Zucchini
- Bottle gourd (*lauki*)
- Ash gourd (*petha*)
- Lettuce
- Spinach (in moderation)
- Broccoli
- Cauliflower

Grains

- Rice (especially basmati)
- Barley
- Wheat
- Oats (when soaked)

Dairy

- Milk (preferably cool, with cardamom)
- Ghee
- Fresh paneer (homemade)
- Buttermilk (with jeera powder)

Herbs and spices

- Fennel
- Mint
- Coriander
- Cardamom
- Sandalwood (external or in beverages)
- Rose (*gulkand* or rose water)

Beverages

- Coconut water
- Fresh sugarcane juice
- Amla juice
- Rose sharbat
- Cumin-coriander-fennel tea

Mechanisms of cooling foods

1. **Regulation of Pitta**: These foods reduce the metabolic heat generated by the Pitta dosha, often through their sweet, bitter or astringent taste and cooling potency.
2. **Hydration**: High water content in foods like watermelon and cucumber aids in heat dissipation through perspiration and urination.
3. **Anti-inflammatory action**: Herbs like coriander and fennel reduce internal inflammation, especially in the gut and skin.
4. **Electrolyte balance**: Natural cooling beverages like coconut water restore the potassium, magnesium and calcium lost via sweat.
5. **Alkalinity**: Many cooling foods help neutralize acidity in the body, reducing heat-related symptoms like acid reflux and burning sensations.

Starting a summer diet

Principles

- Reduce hot and dry foods.
- Focus your diet on moist, cold and sweet-tasting items.

- Avoid overeating; include light, easily digestible meals.
- Emphasize foods with *barid* (cold) and *ratb* (moist) temperament.

Recommended foods

- Barley water
- Tamarind water
- Khus sherbet
- Figs, grapes, pomegranate
- Cucumbers, pumpkins, gourds
- Rose water mixed with milk
- Lettuce, purslane (*kulfa*), spinach
- Lemon and mint juice (shikanji)

Dietary home remedies for increased body heat

1. **Coriander seed water**: Soak one tablespoon of coriander seeds in water overnight. Strain and drink in the morning. Reduces heat and great for acidity, especially skin rashes or burning urine.
2. **Amla juice with honey**: Mix two teaspoons of amla juice with one teaspoon of honey. Take on an empty stomach. Cools the body, rich in vitamin C, supports liver function and Pitta (metabolic) regulation.
3. **Fennel water**: Soak one teaspoon of fennel seeds in water overnight. Strain and drink. Cools the digestive system and reduces acidity. Great drink after giving birth as it regulates motions, reduces flatulence and

increases milk supply. It also relieves colicky babies when consumed through breastmilk.

4. **Coconut water and aloe vera juice**: Mix 1/4 cup aloe vera juice with a glass of coconut water. Extremely cooling and hydrating; helpful for heat-induced headaches or fatigue.
5. **Buttermilk with cumin and mint**: Mix 1/2 cup yogurt with one cup of water, add roasted cumin powder, salt and crushed mint. Aids digestion and cools the gut.
6. **Rose petal jam (gulkand)**: Consume one teaspoon daily, by itself or with milk. A natural refrigerant, it soothes digestive fire and tackles heat boils, acne and burning eyes.

11

OIL AND CHOLESTEROL

'Doctor, is my bad cholesterol high?'

It takes a lot of self-control not to wince every time I hear this question. I feel indignant on behalf of the poor LDL cholesterol; a little flustered because how do I even begin to explain the myth of 'bad' cholesterol? Most of all, frustrated when I end up having to comply with the bad cholesterol terminology so that the patient can better understand my point.

But since we are not pressed for time right now, let me walk you down the cholesterol pathway. We may skip a couple of checkpoints along the way because this ain't a biochemistry textbook but rest assured that we are going to hit all the major milestones.

First things first – LDL isn't cholesterol.

LDL is actually – surprise, surprise – a protein! Specifically, it is a lipoprotein. That means it is a protein entity that transports lipids (fats) in the body, though it does hold some cholesterol, too. There are a few reasons why it is clumped together with cholesterol.

First, it is measured as part of the fasting lipid profile panel. To be clear, this is a measure of lipids rather than cholesterol. However, the two are unfortunately considered the same thing in lay speak. Second, LDL is far easier to temper using drugs than the actual entity that we should be trying to tackle – triglyceride. In fact, statins (the class of medications that lower cholesterol and LDL production) are better tolerated than fenofibrates (medicine that lowers triglycerides). Long story of pharmaceutical manipulation and greed cut short, statins were presented as the drug of choice by lobbyists. The only fault of LDL was that it was more druggable than triglycerides.

A Billion-Dollar Marriage of Convenience

In the mid-1900s, when heart disease was exploding in America, scientists were scrambling for a single villain to blame. After physiologist Ancel Keys stepped forward with a theory that heart disease was caused by fat, the food and pharmaceutical industries saw opportunity. In 1967, sugar industry insiders secretly paid Harvard scientists to publish a highly influential review that downplayed sugar's risks and shifted the blame entirely onto fats – and by extension, LDL cholesterol.[51] There was a public shift to low-fat foods, made palatable by excess sugar. As low-fat, high-sugar products filled supermarket shelves, people's health continued to deteriorate while the industries involved certainly got richer.

The heart disease epidemic refused to relent, even as cholesterol-control guidelines got stricter. The public became sworn enemies of LDL, even though the science was far more nuanced. This set the perfect stage for the rise of statins, drugs designed to lower LDL. Statins quickly became one of the most profitable drug categories in history. And statin was a gift that kept giving because long-time consumers could potentially develop diabetes. A condition whose treatment – you guessed it – was another drug from the same manufacturers!

Only decades later did independent investigations into the sugar lobby reveal behind-the-scenes manipulation, conflicts of interest and how public health advice had been shaped by industry funding rather than unbiased science.[52]

Indiscriminately consuming processed foods, eating when your last meal has not been digested, using refined wheat in your staples – these habits lead to metabolic diseases. It is not the fat in your food that is a bad guy (unless it is trans-fat) but rather freely available glucose. The more you powder your food to dust (maida, I am looking at you), the more carbohydrates get delivered to your system, raising your blood glucose sharply.

Insulin is one hormone that you would die without – it is not a villain. But when you regularly push it to the brink with less-than-ideal eating habits, it does become one.

The carbs you eat – whether in pasta, roti or rice – get converted to glucose. Now insulin has some control issues. You could call it the 'Karen' hormone of your body. Insulin, Karen that she is, ensures the body uses glucose as fuel until there's not much left in the blood. Only then does insulin allow the body to use fat as an energy source. If a person's insulin is high due to regular overeating, their body eventually gets fed up of this bossy hormone and resists its action. This is called, you guessed it, insulin resistance. Here I could explain how insulin resistance wreaks havoc in your body and eventually leads to diabetes. But I shall refrain from taking that route and instead journey to the liver.

The liver has a huge tolerance for insulin. Insulin's home, the pancreas, is the liver's neighbour. So, to simplify things, insulin is more likely to get its way with the liver than the rest of the body. When insulin is high – either because of habitual overeating or insulin resistance as a result of that overeating – the liver is bound to obey its wishes.

Pause.

We need to talk about another bodily process – cholesterol transport.

Fat is absorbed from the intestine in the form of chylomicrons. These are triglycerides wrapped in a molecule called Apo B48. As the chylomicron circulates in the blood it hands out fats to the cells that need them. At a certain point in this journey, the Apo B48 molecule is swapped for Apo 100. With that, the chylomicron transforms into a very-low-density lipoprotein (VLDL).

Lipoproteins are basically a combination of lipid and protein, hence the name. The protein component allows the lipid (fat in simple terms, triglyceride in medical speak) to stay dissolved in the blood instead of floating to the top like butter in churned milk. The density – very-low, low, high – is a marker of how loaded with fat the molecule is. More fat, lower density.

The VLDL eventually transforms into LDL, or low-density lipoprotein. Ideally, this LDL is supposed to go back into your liver and hand off its fat. If needed it is then reassembled and recirculates through the body to supply fat to regenerating and repairing tissues, your endocrine glands for hormone production and all cells which need energy.

Unpause.

Now let's observe how the insulin and cholesterol transport pathways intersect.

The LDL molecule tries to come back to the liver to take a breather before it returns to fuel delivery duty. However, it isn't allowed back into the liver because the organ is too busy handling insulin's tantrum and finding a place to tuck away all the excess glucose from your last binge. The liver stores the glucose in its crevices and lobes in the form of triglycerides. Your liver is like a personal chemistry lab. Glucose to fat, glucose from fat, glucose to protein, glucose from protein – it makes all these conversions possible. The excess glucose that has been tucked away will eventually manifest as fatty liver. It is this fatty liver and high triglycerides that will one day lead you to the doctor's office in low spirits and poor metabolic health, prepared to pop a statin.

Whenever patients inform me that their bad cholesterol is high, the first thing I tell them is that there is no such thing as bad cholesterol. First, cholesterol is good and super important for your body. Cholesterol is the building block of the cell membranes – the covering of each and every cell of your body. It is also the backbone of so many hormones in your body – mainly the sex and adrenal hormones. Secondly, LDL is not even cholesterol! This has been the prank of the century on the public. LDL is a protein that carries fat – it is more protein than we want to admit. The name should be enough of a clue: *low-density* lipoprotein!

In that case, you may wonder, why is LDL always at the crime scene of our clogged arteries?

Triglycerides are produced when three glucose molecules are packaged together with a fatty acid backbone to form a fat molecule. When there is an excess of triglycerides in your body thanks to overconsumption of processed carbs, they will be stored in unusual places. This is the origin of the fatty streaks in your arteries that will one day progress to a full-on blockade. LDL is just doing its job: carrying the triglyceride molecule and wandering your blood in search of a cell that will accept this overdose of fuel.

Also, there are two types of LDL: small, dense (sdLDL) and large, buoyant (lbLDL). The lbLDL is affected by dietary fat (so it reduces when you improve your diet) and cholesterol-lowering medication. Out of the total LDL measured, this type accounts for a three-fourth majority. But here is the catch: lbLDL cholesterol does not clog your arteries!

The sdLDL is the true Shakuni mama in your lipid reports. They are small, conniving and bad for your heart health. Science is still not a 100 per cent sure how bad sdLDL is for you but it is abundantly clear that high levels of sdLDL mean a greater risk of heart disease and heart attacks. Unfortunately, even if sdLDL is just a quarter of your total LDL, the reports don't tell us how much of each kind is elevated.

I hope it's becoming clear that the solution to your health woes isn't as simple as 'lowering cholesterol'. Think of it this way. You need glasses but don't wear them. This means you get a headache nearly every day. So, what do you do? You keep taking paracetamol daily to get rid of the ache. Have you treated the easily manageable headache with glasses? No, not yet. But you are 'treating' the headache with pain medicine nonetheless.

The same applies here. There is a false, misdirected sense of urgency to 'treat' your cholesterol. In actuality, it's your improper diet and lack of activity that needs fixing. It's the overflooding of your body with fuel that needs to be curtailed. Once you take these steps, insulin resistance will diminish over time and your fatty liver will become just a liver, your fatty pancreas will be just a pancreas and your LDL can do its work in peace without being bulldozed by excess insulin or labelled bad. But coming to this realization in today's world is an uphill battle because LDL is druggable, drugs cost money and big pharma isn't willing to give that up. And don't forget that these companies both influence the studies which very lopsidedly support all data speaking in favour of their drugs and sponsor the medical institutions that teach your doctors. The question isn't whether the pharma chicken or doctor's egg came first. Big pharma is the chicken as well as the egg. They have a huge say in setting your doctor's education and treatment protocol. So this isn't your doctor's fault either!

Now that I have got LDL out of the way, let's briefly speak about cholesterol. For the most part, it does not come from food but the liver. There, I said it!

The cholesterol we consume is only minimally absorbed by the intestine. No matter what you do to 'reduce dietary cholesterol', your liver will continue to manufacture this crucial molecule. The only way to stop this process is by throwing a drug into your body and in most cases, that isn't necessary. Fun fact: researchers have estimated that life expectancy for statin users increases by a mere ten days over a six-year period.[53] [54] That's it. Just ten days! Yet authorities like the American Heart Association endorse statin therapy as the first-line treatment for those with heart disease risk factors. By that criterion, we are all candidates.

Oil, Villain and Victim

It is sad to see people these days boiling their veggies before gobbling them down in haste. Haste because it tastes so bland and our tongues hate bland. My mission with this book is to encourage you to eat in sync with the cycle of nature and your body. Nothing good has ever come of villainizing an entire food group. I have to admit that I wouldn't mind seeing processed food taken to task but I have a feeling many industrialists will be pissed off if that were to happen.

Oil is essential to life. It is a rich source of brain-building molecules, a *suraksha kawach* for our skin, a carrier of precious vitamins. Perhaps most importantly, it is the tastemaker of our food. For the longest time, oil was our medium of choice when preparing food. Until the late twentieth century, when experts suddenly began pressuring us to go fat-free.

The reality is that the fat in your belly is not the same as the fat in your food. In this section, I plan to debunk some common misconceptions about oil consumption. And as a bonus, I will talk about how the nature of your oil changes when you apply it externally. Trust me, your body is going to love you for smearing this greasy goodness on it!

For instance, it was long believed that the brain was untouched by insulin – that it would be fuelled by glucose irrespective of whether your pancreas worked. However, recent studies have shown that there are insulin dependent receptors in the brain. These receptors are for brain and memory function, not energy uptake.

So, what happens when your body is flooded with insulin because of insulin resistance? The brain starts to reel, particularly when there is high insulin and normal blood sugar as seen in the early stages of metabolic diseases. Eventually, this translates to poor memory, dementia and even Alzheimer's disease. It was found that the plaques of Alzheimer's disease were more common in areas where insulin receptors are the highest.[55] Don't worry, you are not going to lose your memory overnight because you have borderline or even overt diabetes. In addition to lifestyle modification and increased activity, an unexpected ingredient – oil – might be able to help you combat insulin resistance. Spoiler alert: no one oil suits all.

If you are wondering what oil to opt for because the tropical city you live in feels temperate thanks to the AC, worry not. Respect your genetic makeup and the science of nutrigenomics – stick to the oil you and your ancestors have grown up consuming. However, it's possible that you grew up with a cosmopolitan, confused kitchen that featured new oils every second month. After all, mothers across generations have had to keep up with diet fads, albeit less than what we face now. In that case, revert to the food's temperament. Having idli, sambhar and chutney for breakfast? Go for coconut oil in the tadka. Shivering because of the winter chill? Stir fry your mutton in sesame oil. Thinking of snacking on hummus? Add a splash of olive oil. These oils are the perfect carriers for the good molecules of spices *and* make your food taste better. So don't sauté your food in water as some Insta influencers will tell you to and choose oil instead.

Coconut oil – nourishing India's most literate state

The humble *nariyal tel* which our mothers massaged into our scalps before washing our hair is now quite the talk of the town. One day it is the hero you need in your food, coffee, toothpaste and hair conditioner. The next year it faces a witch trial, accused of being replete with 'bad' fats. The following year it is a hero once again. This cycle has repeated ad nauseum over the last three decades. The main reason why coconut oil finds itself embroiled in controversy despite its goodness – known to humans for centuries – is its fatty acid content. It is rich in saturated fats.

Oh, the horror.

I have said it before and I will say it again: saturated fats aren't bad for you. Saturated fats don't clog your arteries; unlimited fuel intake does. In fact, they have a nice silver lining. Since they don't have a double bond, saturated fats cannot convert to trans fats.

The MCFAs and monoglycerides from coconut are absorbed in the small intestine. These free fatty acids fuel the body directly because they do not need to be metabolized further through degradation and esterification. And as a cherry on top, they are not deposited as fat in the body.

Another awesome thing about coconut oil is that its MCFA content gets converted to ketones in the liver.

(All those on the keto diet bandwagon, don't celebrate just yet). These ketones travel to the insulin receptors in the brain to prevent the formation of Alzheimer's plaques and preserve brain function. In growing babies, applying coconut oil to their head and body helps hasten weight gain (crucial for premature babies) and brain development.[56,57] One study followed a sample of babies for a year to study this link. Those who received coconut oil massages reached their neurodevelopmental milestones earlier. The exact mechanism hasn't yet been fully understood but several theories have been proposed. The oil may create a protective barrier that reduces infections and the deep stimulating touch tempers episodes of apnoea so babies grow better. Some of the fatty acids are absorbed through the skin and into the bloodstream. This extra supply of fats supports weight gain and rapid brain growth, contributing to earlier milestone achievement.[58]

Coconut and the gut

Coconut oil increases the composition of good bacteria in the gut. This leads to better metabolism, less deposition of fat on organs and fewer cravings. The lauric acid composition of coconut oil helps nourish the *Lactobacillus* and *Bifidobacterium* bacteria in the gut which in turn reduce the population of bad bacteria and provide a big metabolic advantage.

Gastric trouble is one of the most common complaints I hear in my practice. Indiscriminately using antacids is only a temporary salve that does not address underlying issues. Heavy smoking, excessive caffeine consumption or an undiagnosed *H. pylori* infection can wreak havoc in your stomach lining and causes ulcers. Virgin coconut oil works wonders for addressing all these pathologies.

In fact, gastric ulcers or even simple gastritis caused by overuse of painkillers respond better to virgin coconut oil when compared to arguably the best antacid available – omeprazole. Where omeprazole indiscriminately lowers acid production, coconut oil has a more beneficial holistic action. Think of this scenario. When public outrage occurs because of some gross injustice, the omeprazole government would call for curfews and curb internet access. Whereas the virgin coconut oil government would reassure the grieving public and tackle the issue that sparked the uproar.

Even though coconut oil has a cooling nature, it strengthens digestive Agni. It does so without compromising the important acid-producing function of the stomach. The gastric juice produced by virgin coconut oil has much lower total acidity and ulcer-causing potential. It tends to the disrupted mucus barrier of the stomach and has an antibacterial effect against the *H. pylori* bacteria. Coconut oil also increases protective factors in the stomach lining such as nitrites and glutathione (GSH). GSH is very crucial for overall gut health as it protects the cells against toxic injury. This is invaluable as we take in a *lot* of toxins via the gut route. Just think of Saturday night – *chakhna* and booze galore.

Coconut oil also reduces the action of prostaglandins and has been shown to reduce period cramps. Just apply some coconut oil on your lower abdomen if you want to avoid the Meftal Spas.

The new mother

After childbirth, women undergo major hormonal shifts that affect mood, energy and overall well-being. Coconut oil, rich in lauric acid and MCFAs, supports stress responses and thyroid function. Lauric acid helps modulate the hypothalamic-pituitary-adrenal axis and reduces stress-related cortisol, while the fats provide energy, enhance mitochondrial activity and aid in converting the thyroid hormone T4 to its active form T3.

At the same time, the new mother's doshas shift significantly. Vata is the most aggravated, leading to restlessness, anxiety, dry skin and irregular sleep. Pitta may rise slightly, causing irritability, hot flashes or a tendency for skin flare-ups. Kapha on the other hand is depleted because ... well, she made a baby. This translates to low immunity and fatigue. A warm coconut oil massage addresses all three – it grounds Vata, soothes Pitta and restores Kapha. Thus, it offers holistic support for hormonal balance, stress regulation and postpartum recovery.

Sesame oil – queen of seed oils

Sesame oil is warm in nature and helps balance Vata and Kapha. Coconuts are traditionally grown and consumed in tropical regions where the weather is hot for most of the year. Thus, the local population benefits from its cooling nature. In contrast, sesame grows predominantly in dry, temperate regions and is a good addition to your winter diet. Sesame oil is used just like coconut oil – a cooking medium, hair oil, skin moisturizer and for the practice of oil pulling to maintain oral hygiene. Tahini, made from sesame seeds, is a wonder food for lactating mothers (you might remember this from the chapter on hot foods).

Sesame is replete with omega-3, omega-6 and omega-9, providing a balance between all the essential fatty acids. Sesame has a mild laxative effect that pacifies Vata. The lignan composition of this oil ensures smooth bowel movements every day and prevents gas build-up, bloating and constipation. Sesame lignans also influence the body's metabolism. True to its Kapha-improving function, sesame oil checks the fatty liver, reduces cholesterol and protects against diabetes and high BP. A note of caution, overdosing on sesame oil will worsen Kapha. Balance is key. Sauté your veggies and deep fry only once in a while.

The mechanism by which sesame oil reduces cholesterol is the same as the highest-selling cholesterol-lowering medication – statins. Both inhibit the enzyme HMG-CoA reductase but the God-made sesame does come with a little dose of divinity. When consumed in moderation (just like any oil should be), it saves you from high cholesterol levels and clogged arteries without the side effects of statins – myopathy (muscle loss) and dementia (memory loss). In fact, statins increase the risk of depression and suicide when taken long term, particularly when started at a young age.[59] 25 per cent of your body's cholesterol is in the brain, imperative for its functioning. Statins disrupt that. Not on sesame oil's watch!

According to TCM, sesame seeds nourish our internal organs and replenish marrow. A component of sesame oil called sesamin promotes osteoblastic differentiation of bone marrow stromal cells. In simpler words, it increases bone density and protects against age-related bone weakening (osteoporosis). Elderly women often suffer from osteoporosis due to decreased oestrogen after menopause. Even minor falls and bumps can lead to fractured bones. Sesame oil is the perfect choice if you want to reclaim your bone health at menopause.

Rheumatoid arthritis is a chronic multi-system autoimmune disease. In Ayurveda, joint disease is generally attributed to an imbalance of Vata. The hallmark finding in this disease is persistent and progressive joint destruction. Since the body's immune system is mounting an inappropriate response against itself, the main line of treatment in contemporary medicine is suppressing the immune system on the body level as well as locally at the joint level.

Painkillers such as Diclofenac and Ibuprofen are often prescribed to soothe joint pain and swelling. Unfortunately, with long-term use, these drugs can cause side effects such as stomach ulcers, kidney damage and a bleeding tendency.

Another line of treatment is the use of steroids. Again, these powerful drugs can spawn a host of adverse effects. Long-term use of glucocorticoids can give the patient stomach ulcers, high BP, weakened bones and compromise their immunity. Disease-modifying antirheumatoid drugs (DMARDs) are a mainstay for treating arthritis but they too are fraught with so many side effects. Chronic use can suppress bone marrow and cause non-healing mouth ulcers, baldness and diarrhoea. They can also reduce the patient's blood platelet count, potentially triggering organ toxicity and a bleeding tendency.

An ideal drug for this debilitating lifelong disease has been in dire demand. Studies have shown that sesame oil's efficacy is comparable to the most-prescribed drugs – methotrexate (a DMARD) and diclofenac (an anti-inflammatory). Even though the research is quite nascent, it has raised a lot of hope. Not only did sesame oil relieve pain and swelling but also the joints showed remarkable improvement compared to conventional drugs. In a way, these drugs indiscriminately block the pathology and do little to improve or reverse the condition. On the other hand, sesame oil works on all fronts and helps improve the disease pathology.

Every single phytonutrient present in sesame oil contributes to improving the underlying processes at play in rheumatoid arthritis. It is astonishing how adeptly sesame oil handles the full body effects of this disease. Rheumatoid arthritis is often accompanied by anaemia and TCM practitioners were right when they said sesame 'fills' the marrow. By prompting the bone marrow to produce more red blood cells and platelets, it precludes the need for additional drugs to treat anaemia. Its ability to increase red blood cell numbers and counter a Vata condition make it the quintessential 'hot' oil.

As I write this section I have a knee injury. I dislocated my kneecap while doing yoga – a ligament injury. I have been applying a pain relief oil on my knee every night. It has a comforting warmth and relieves the stiffness in my joint, since I keep my leg straightened in a brace all day long. When I looked at the ingredient list of the magical oil, the first component happened to be, you guessed it, sesame oil!

This treatment is yet to have a standardized dose or be adopted into Western medicine. In the meantime, apply warm sesame oil on your joints and use it in your daily cooking to reap its benefits.

Gingelly oil – the elixir of youth

Gingelly oil is Indian sesame oil. Extracted at a high temperature, it is amber in colour and has a low smoking point. It is safe for cooking but best avoided when deep frying. Sesame oil, on the contrary, is pale yellow and extracted through the cold press method. The high smoke point of sesame oil makes it ideal for deep frying, too.

Just like our hardy coconut oil, gingelly oil is a great skincare remedy. It rapidly penetrates the skin's basal layer and provides deep moisture. It protects the skin against sun damage and reduces fine lines and wrinkles. In fact, one could called it an anti-ageing oil. It is very effective at attracting and eroding oil-soluble pollutants. When applied to the skin, the pollutants disperse in the oil and are wiped away.

Gingelly oil also has numerous benefits when applied to the hair. It has hair-darkening characteristics and prevents greying. It is an excellent deep purifier for hair, restores hair strength and prevents hairfall. Just like sesame oil, it protects the joints and preserves mobility. Luscious black hair, smooth supple skin and strong joints – gingelly oil is the elixir of youth.

The oil is rich in copper, which makes it an excellent candidate for herbal relief salves for joint pain. Irrespective of the cause of arthritis, the Vata dosha is pacified by applying gingelly oil. Copper helps normalize anti-inflammatory and antioxidant enzymatic reactions, significantly lowering arthritic discomfort and pain. Copper also enhances blood vessel strength and increases joint and bone density.

Zinc deficiency may lead to osteoporosis or the fracturing of bone fragments in the spine and hips. The oil contains zinc, which induces skeletal wellness and bone mineral density. Finally, in case you needed further convincing about its useful properties, gingelly oil has high calcium content.

Sweet almond oil – the superficial laxative

Warming like sesame, sweet almond oil is the medicine you should turn to in case of gas and constipation. Even better news, you just have to massage your tummy with it. One study compared the effect of almond oil on gut mobility when ingested or massaged as opposed to no intervention. The results showed that using the oil – whether consumed or massaged on the belly – was linked to a significant improvement in quality of life due to built-up waste being cleared out of the subject's body.[60]

Here's how to relieve yourself of gas and constipation *without* gulping down a laxative:

- Before you start the massage, make sure both the oil and your hands are warm – warm, not hot. Rub your hands together for half a minute before touching the belly. This will ensure the abdominal wall is sufficiently relaxed. Touch a belly with cold hands and it will reflexively tighten up!
- Stroke upwards from the belly button towards the breastbone to relax the abdominal muscles. In case of a history of hiatus hernia or acid reflux, stroke downwards instead. This action helps relax the abdominal muscle.
- Start your gentle massage from the lower back and gradually move forward over the flank on either side to stimulate the vagus nerve. This will tell the bowel to wake up. Then stroke from the small (centre) of your back, round and down the crease of the hip

bones on either side and end at the groin. Repeat ten times.

- The next massage stroke is called effleurage. Use the palms of your hands and stroke the abdomen with light pressure in a clockwise direction for two minutes. This will move faecal matter along and stimulate bowel movement.
- The heat of the massage and kneading helps propel faeces along the colon to load the rectum. Use gentle but firm pressure with your palms for this stage of the massage.
- Knead the left side of the abdomen downwards, as this is where the descending colon lies. Continue for two minutes. Follow this with two minutes of upward palmar kneading on the right side, waking up the ascending colon. Now return to the left side and repeat the palmar kneading for another two minutes.
- Repeat the effleurage step for another two minutes.
- End the massage with ten gentle strokes to relax your abdominal muscles and help your body understand that the massage is ending. Finally, gently drum your fingers over the navel for a minute to relieve wind.

This massage can be done using sesame oil too. I would not recommend drinking sesame or almond oil for constipation relief as they can interfere with BP medication and even lower BP to the point of fainting. The massage is a safer approach until the interaction between the oils and common medicines used by the elderly is established scientifically. Just make sure to use gentle firm pressure and remain cautious in case of a preexisting hernia.

Castor oil – hot or cold?

Writing about this oil has been the hardest part of the chapter. Castor oil has long been prized for promoting long, luscious hair and, in alternative medicine, inducing labour. Its famous laxative and labour-inducing effects make it the quintessential hot oil.

So, what was my conundrum?

I once met a patient whose hair was striking – beautiful, dark, long; straight with no evidence of ever having being touched by a straightener. During the consultation, she mentioned that her sinuses became blocked every time she applied hair oil. She used a base of coconut oil and added castor oil and a few drops of rosemary oil. Fresh from my research on essential oils, I told her to not use rosemary oil.

After the consult I spoke to my coordinator about the patient, smug that I was able to apply my newfound knowledge. My coordinator, more well-versed with the nature of castor oil, immediately corrected me. Castor oil has a hot nature when ingested, causing the gut and uterus to contract. This is a testament to its Vata-pacifying action. Simply put, the oil gets things moving out of your body. However, though it is predominantly Vata-pacifying, castor oil also has a gentle Kapha-modulating action. For a Kapha-predominant person, it can tip the balance and cause sinus congestion when applied topically. Thus, the distinction between hot and cold becomes a little blurry – the so-called cooling effect is Kapha promotion and the hot effect is Vata promotion. Hang in there, this will become clearer in the following paragraphs.

Castor oil has a remarkable ability to be absorbed by the skin, making it a top choice for enhancing hair growth. By countering dryness (a Vata issue) and improving nutrient transport (also a Vata issue), it nourishes the scalp and hair follicles deeply. Its thick consistency allows the oil to penetrate the layers of the skin and reach the follicles, revitalizing dormant roots, encouraging new growth and reducing hair loss.[61] The main fatty acid in castor oil, ricinoleic acid, is responsible for its unique therapeutic properties.[62] Ricinoleic acid calms scalp inflammation and dryness (goodbye, dandruff!) while the vitamin E, proteins and omega-6 fatty acids contained by the oil nourish the roots and scalp.

Castor oil's generosity is not limited to the superficial; its benefits extend to the intricate ECM that supports and feeds hair follicle cells.[63] A quick recap here – ECM maintenance is the Kapha dosha's department. The matrices are fortified by the fatty acids present in castor oil. It breathes new life into the hair follicle cells by rejuvenating the ECM, resulting in the growth of longer, sturdier strands. Moreover, castor oil boasts qualities that positively impact the ground regulatory system, a crucial player in hair cycling. As hair follicles transition through various phases of growth and rest in their life cycle, castor oil steps in to maintain a delicate balance.

An ode to TCM

According to TCM, the body's organs are interconnected and influenced by the principles of yin and yang. Yin organs (*zang*) are solid and store vital substances like blood and essence, while yang organs (*fu*) are hollow and responsible for transforming and transporting fluids and food, maintaining the body's functions. Applying this perspective to castor oil's effects, we can explore its impact on the colon and lungs.

The colon, a yang organ, is vital for waste elimination and regulating the body's water balance. Castor oil's purgative properties help stimulate bowel movement and waste removal from the colon. This cleansing action aligns with TCM's concept of eliminating excess yang energy and restoring balance to the body's systems.

Conversely, the lungs, classified as a yin organ, are responsible for respiration and maintaining the body's vitality through the intake of oxygen. Castor oil's soothing properties (Vata pacification) alleviate inflammation and congestion in the respiratory system. As TCM puts it, castor oil supports lung function and overall respiratory health by reducing excess heat and promoting a harmonious flow of energy.

Though this might sound like pseudoscience, it is backed by science entirely! Studies show that ricinoleic acid's anti-inflammatory effect calms irritated airways, leading to reduced mucus secretion and airway reactivity. This is very useful for patients experiencing chest congestion, as seen in asthma and bronchitis. Lymphatic flow is also enhanced, clearing toxins and fluid build-up that often worsen congestion.

Coming back to TCM, the colon and lungs are considered paired organs that influence each other's functioning. Addressing imbalances in one organ, such as promoting bowel regularity with castor oil, positively impacts the health of its pair. We see this action at play when castor oil is administered to newborns – a common, time-tested practice in Indian homes that is now shunned by modern medicine.

I was a puritan practitioner of Western medicine when my first kid was born, so I kept castor oil far away from him. His dadi wanted to give him a drop or two of castor oil to help clear out the blackish tarry stools that are typical of newborns. She told me it was great for the baby's gut and would protect against chest congestion. According to traditional wisdom, the latter outlasts castor oil's temporary local effect on the colon. Of course, I stood my ground and didn't allow it to happen.

I approached castor oil with a newfound sense of humility and openness when my second kid was born, having witnessed a few episodes of childhood bronchitis in my son. As her dadi had predicted, she remained remarkably resilient despite being in contact with her older brother when he was sick. This could potentially be attributed both to exclusive breastfeeding and the occasional use of castor oil.

Like all remedies, castor oil has the rare side effect if taken in high doses. My paediatrician warned me against using it because it could potentially cause gastrointestinal upset. However, in my experience, it has effectively relieved constipation and chest congestion in my son.

Across India, families have historically used castor oil for newborns in various ways, usually guided by grandmothers and midwives. Bear in mind that this guidance is only meant for traditional home-remedy use – not as a paediatric medical prescription. A lick of castor oil was routinely given to newborns to 'clean the stomach' – a reference to the tarry first stools of a newborn. My mother-in-law, for instance, would simply let the baby lick the faint smear of castor oil that clung to her fingertip – never an actual drop. This practice was followed every alternate day for the first two weeks when taking the baby for their daily sunbath.

Castor oil is best consumed first thing in the morning on an empty stomach. It should always be warmed slightly before giving it to a child and used with caution – never during fever or active respiratory infections. A child weighing around ten kilograms generally needs no more than half a teaspoon of warmed oil. My own children typically received castor oil once every two to three months until they were about five to six years old – enough to enjoy its traditional benefits while minimizing risk.

Rosemary oil – the hijabi's secret

The secret behind many a hijabi girl's surprisingly luscious mane? Not expensive treatments, just rosemary oil. This humble herb has been a beauty favourite across the Middle East and Mediterranean for generations, long before TikTok rediscovered it. Used for centuries, it has a reputation for strengthening roots, stimulating growth and keeping hair healthy despite heat and covering hair.

As per both TCM and Ayurveda, rosemary (*Rujamari* in India) is thought to have a warm or stimulating nature. It promotes Pitta by generating a stimulating effect on circulation. When applied topically or inhaled, its aromatic compounds dilate blood vessels, increase blood flow and provide a feeling of warmth. Try to apply this knowledge to your winter hair care routine. Warm coconut oil with a few drops of rosemary essential oil makes for a great night-time scalp massage. Use gentle pressure and have a head bath after thirty minutes or in the morning.

Rosmarinic acid, one of the antioxidant compounds in rosemary oil, helps protect against oxidative damage and rejuvenate the ECM. Rife with anti-inflammatory and antioxidant compounds which modulate immune cell activity, it tempers the production of pro-inflammatory cytokines in the scalp tissue. Scalp inflammation often shows up as itching, redness, flaking, tenderness or a burning sensation. This inflammation weakens the roots and further triggers hair fall. Rosemary oil also prolongs the growth phase of hair (anagen), reducing hair loss and promoting growth.[64]

While rosemary oil is generally considered safe for topical use, do a patch test to check for skin sensitivities before applying it to your scalp. Just because it is natural does not mean it won't prompt an allergic reaction. Thousands of people around the world are deathly allergic to peanuts, after all. Additionally, consult a dermatologist ahead of using the oil if you have any underlying scalp or hair conditions.

An essential thing to know about essential oils is that they are extremely volatile. Apply them in isolation and they will evaporate into thin air before you know it. Even worse, they might cause skin irritation. Oils such as rosemary or lavender should always be used after mixing in a base oil - coconut is your best bet. Use about two to three drops of rosemary oil per tablespoon of carrier oil. And do not - I repeat, do *not* - dilute an essential oil with another essential oil!

The most fitting conclusion to this discussion on oil is reiterating the importance of modulation in alternate medicine. When the recommended dose of a food / food group / herb / herbal formulation is taken, it works to modulate the cell, ECM and circulation supplying that tissue. Just like us humans, cells are not independent. We need family (cells that form a tissue), society (tissues that form an organ) and meaningful societal relationships (circulation and connection to major blood vessels). A healthy cell lives in a healthy matrix with healthy circulation. Depending on your innate and current doshic nature, you need to adjust your meals, meal timings and lifestyle, including exercise.

This principle of modulation is at the heart of traditional medicine. Many home remedies are not quick fixes. Instead, they gently steer the body back towards balance using everyday ingredients. With this understanding, we can now explore how simple household practices – from oils to spices to kitchen staples – restore health by supporting rather than overwhelming the body's natural intelligence.

12

REMEDIES FROM THE KITCHEN

> 'Medicine is preservation of health and restoring it when it gets lost'
>
> IBN SINA, Father of Modern Medicine

In this chapter, we're taking a walk back into the kitchen because sometimes the simplest ingredients can do far more than flavour our food. Across generations, people have reached for turmeric, ginger, honey, ajwain and dozens of other everyday items to calm infections, ease discomfort and support healing. These remedies weren't created in labs; they were developed out of observation, common sense, intuition and a deep understanding of how the body responds to nature. Here, we revisit that wisdom in a practical, modern way.

You'll notice that the chapter is arranged by body system – respiratory, digestive, metabolic, skin and hair, and so on. Yes, the body doesn't always behave in clean compartments. A 'digestive issue' can easily show up on your skin, while a 'respiratory issue' may start in the gut. Still, this simple structure will make it easier to find what you need quickly.

Traditional home remedies naturally blend both worlds: they help mitigate symptoms and gently address the underlying imbalances that caused them in the first place. The remedies in this chapter are meant to support you, not replace proper medical care. They work beautifully as additions to your routine but they're not substitutes for a doctor's diagnosis, prescribed treatment or emergency care.

Fever

Indications: High body temperature, physical pain, fatigue

Fever is the body's natural response to infection, triggered by the immune system to hinder pathogens. While mild to moderate fever (up to 102 degrees Fahrenheit or 38.9 degrees Celsius) can be managed with rest and hydration, higher temperatures require medical attention to prevent complications.

Tulsi (holy basil)

Directions: Boil two teaspoons of tulsi powder or a fistful of fresh tulsi leaves in 100 ml of water for five minutes. Sip warm. Repeat three to four times a day until symptoms reduce.

Respiratory System

Seasonal flu and cold

Indications: Cold, cough with watery phlegm
Directions: Mix 20 g of black seeds (kalonji) with 50 g long pepper powder (pippali). Not to be confused with clove (laung) or black peppercorn (kali mirch)! Consume 5 g of this mixture twice a day, one hour after breakfast and dinner. Continue this course for three to four days.

Avoid taking large doses if you are about to undergo a surgery. High amounts of kalonji reduce the clotting capacity of blood which can lead to internal bleeds. These seeds need to be limited to very small quantities.

Tonsillitis

Indications: Fever, cough, throat pain

Qust refers to the dried root of *Saussurea costus* or the costus root. There are two varieties: Qust al-Hind (Indian costus) and Qust al-Bahri (sea incense). Hot and dry by nature, both help combat phlegm and colds.

Not only does costus help reduce the viral load in the body but it is also effective against multidrug-resistant bacteria. Tonsillitis with high fever? Qust al-Bahri powder mixed with honey will make your tonsils feel better. But your tastebuds ... not so much. I almost gagged the first time I tried it.

Directions: Combine the powdered root with honey and thin the mixture further with water. Also ensure your vitamin D levels are healthy for proper mineral absorption. Adults can consume 5 g of raw costus daily, ideally post breakfast or dinner. Continue for ten to twelve days. Adapt the dose for children aged three to eight (2 g) and nine to fifteen (½ teaspoon).

Avoid if allergic to Asteraceae plants (e.g., daisy, dandelion). Children under three and pregnant or breastfeeding mothers should steer clear due to limited research. Indian costus may contain aristolochic acid, which is toxic to kidneys and carcinogenic in excess. There are strict laws in place to ensure aristolochic acid-free products but contamination can occur if members of the Aristolochia species are misidentified or substituted for *Saussurea costus*, the true source of Qust al-Hind.

Breathing problems

Indications: Thick phlegm, wheezing, asthma

Kalonji contains a chemical compound called nigellone which prevents histamine release from mast cells. This targets the root cause of airway hyper-reactivity, making it an effective tool to combat asthma. It reduces secretions and relaxes airways. A three-month study showed improved lung function in asthmatic patients who were consuming boiled kalonji extract.[65]

Directions: Mix 5 g of kalonji powder with one teaspoon of honey. Eat this paste twice a day, one hour after breakfast and dinner. Continue for three to four days. This remedy works as an expectorant and gives relief from chest congestion. A more chronic episode would require a personalized dietary plan for the patient.

Allergic sinusitis

Indications: Nasal congestion, sneezing, facial pressure, watery eyes

Allergic sinusitis is a sign of an overactive immune response. Avoiding the allergen is the best treatment but often we cannot pinpoint a singular cause. What starts as an irritation that might prevent you from getting a good night's rest can turn into a long-standing dry cough if treated only with drying antihistaminics. A simple cinnamon-based home remedy may help prevent this.

Directions: Add two cinnamon sticks or 5 g of cinnamon powder to 250 ml water. Boil for five minutes. Add a pinch of turmeric powder and honey. Drink once a day, one hour before eating. Can be taken for a week.

Nervous System

Anxiety and palpitations

Today we are connected to millions of people online yet live very isolated lives. As community living gradually disappears, we are all our own islands, drifting away from one another. Hustle culture, crippling anxiety and soul-sucking depression; sleeplessness, dependency on social media and the weight of work pressure. If these experiences sound familiar, there is a humble home remedy for your nerves waiting to be discovered.

Quince (safarjal) is a pear-like fruit that Unani describes as a *Mufarrih* – food that uplifts the spirit. Its mild sedative and anxiolytic action calms the autonomic nervous system. It helps improve vagal tone so your body can prioritize rest and digestion over the flight or fight state typical in anxiety. This leads to a lower resting heart rate and fewer episodes of anxiety-related palpitations. The phenolics and flavonoids in quince modulate serotonin and GABA levels, important for mood regulation.

Directions: Wash and cut the quince into small pieces. Retain the skin but remove the seeds. Boil in water for about fifteen to twenty minutes until soft. Let it cool, then mash the pulp and mix in honey and three to four strands of saffron (optional). Consume warm in the morning or after dinner, three to four times a week.

Sciatica

Indications: Pain in the lower back, buttocks, legs

Sciatica is pain that travels along the path of the sciatic nerve, the longest nerve in the body. It begins in the lower back, runs through the buttocks and branches down each leg. Though not a disease itself, sciatica is symptomatic of an underlying condition. It usually happens when something compresses or irritates the sciatic nerve – spinal issues, muscle spasms, tumours, infections or physical trauma. Pain management and physiotherapy can help. Nerve pain is considered an outcome of Vata disturbance, so foods which improve Vata – warm, oily, nourishing, grounding – are recommended for sciatica too. Avoid dry, cold and gas-producing items (e.g., raw salads, legumes, aerated drinks, brinjal).

Spice therapy

Separately grind 10 g ginger, 5 g black pepper, 10 g turmeric, 15 g fenugreek seeds and 5 g garlic. Mix and store in an airtight container. Consume 5 g (one teaspoon) on an empty stomach in the morning and another one hour after dinner. Take for two weeks followed by a week-long break. Continue this cycle.

Sheep tail fat

Fat-tailed sheep are a domestic variety characterized by their large tails and behinds. As per prophetic medicine, tail fat from such sheep is a remedy for sciatica and nerve pain. Sheep tail fat is thought to calm the Vata dosha, which corresponds to nerve hyperactivity. The tallow nourishes the spine and joints when consumed or applied. It is rich in conjugated linoleic acid (CLA), fat-soluble vitamins (A, D, K) and saturated fats, which help support the nerves and control inflammation.

To prepare the tallow:

1. Use tail fat from grass-fed, pasture-raised sheep only. Good-quality fat is key.
2. Remove the meat, blood clots and connective tissue. Chop the fat into small cubes.

3. Now dry render the fat. Place it in a heavy-bottomed pot over low heat, stirring occasionally until it melts and separates. The fat will turn into golden liquid while solids (cracklings) float to the surface.
4. Strain through a clean cotton cloth while hot. Store in a glass jar. Let it cool until it solidifies into creamy-white tallow.
5. The tallow will last several months if kept cool and dry. Refrigeration is preferred.

Directions: Take one to two teaspoons daily, on an empty stomach in the morning or with warm water/milk at night. Combine with a pinch of kalonji or ajwain powder for an added anti-inflammatory effect. Use for seven to twenty-one days, depending on symptom severity.

Optionally, you can also apply the tallow topically. Warm it gently and massage it over the lower back, hips or sciatic path at night.

Avoid during active liver infections, gallbladder disease or if you're on a strict low-fat diet. Sheep tail fat is a food adjunct and not a substitute for surgery or clinical intervention if nerve compression is severe.

Sleep disturbance

Indications: Depression, anxiety, hyperactive mind, general weakness

Pumpkin seeds

Pumpkin seeds have a sedating effect that makes them an excellent sleep aid without the accompanying dependence we often see with sleeping pills. They are rich in the amino acid tryptophan – the precursor of sleep hormones serotonin and melatonin.

Eat two tablespoons of roasted pumpkin seeds an hour before bed to support melatonin production.

Barley-based talbina

Barley's natural fibres feed the good gut bacteria that produce calming, GABA-boosting compounds – the same chemistry your brain uses to wind down at night. Barley also contains tryptophan, the building block your body uses to make serotonin and melatonin, the hormones that help you fall asleep and stay asleep. And because barley is a slow, gentle carb, it keeps your blood sugar steady, which in turn keeps evening cortisol in check. Lower cortisol means your nervous system can slip into the relaxed, rest-and-digest state you need for restorative sleep.

Best eaten during breakfast and dinner. Those who are sick can consume it three to four times a day. Refer to Chapter 10 for the recipe!

Digestive System

Acid reflux

Indications: Acidity, heartburn, hot sensation in the stomach

Nabeez

It is a drink prepared by soaking raisins, figs or dates in water overnight and drinking the mixture in the morning. This method makes the antioxidant content of the fruits more available to the body for absorption. For acid reflux, raisin-based nabeez is an excellent choice.

Directions: Add two teaspoons of golden raisins to a glass of water and let them soak overnight. Consume the water and raisins on an empty stomach the following morning. You can have breakfast after an hour-long gap.

Avoid for diabetic patients. Soak only in glass or earthen utensils.

Black seeds

Research has shown that black seed oil – thanks to its key compound thymoquinone – can fight *H. pylori*, the bacteria often linked to hyperacidity and stomach ulcers. It works almost as well as the standard triple-drug therapy for people with heartburn (but no ulcers). It protects the stomach by reducing excess acid and histamines that can irritate the stomach. It also boosts natural defences like mucin (the stomach's protective lining) and glutathione (an antioxidant).

Directions: Add a spoonful of kalonji to your dough when making rotis, parathas or puris – elevating the flavour while imbibing its benefits. You can also make a panchphoran (*panch* = five, *phoran* = tempering) mix, best used as a tadka for sabzis. This mix works as a great carminative and digestive. It is particularly helpful for the postpartum period as it reduces gas and increases breastmilk supply. I make a mean cauliflower sabzi with just this tempering, ginger garlic paste and basic spice powders. The gas formation because of the cauliflower is offset by these tiny seeds.

Constipation

Indications: Constipation, bloated stomach

Fig-based nabeez

Soak figs in water overnight. In the morning, grind along with water and consume on an empty stomach. Continue the course for a week or two for best results.

Sana makki

Also known as senna or *Cassia angustifolia*, sana makki is a herb commonly used in traditional medicine – particularly in Unani Tibb. Primarily the leaves and sometimes the pods are utilized for medicinal purposes, often in tea or capsule form. Like other varieties of senna, the herb is renowned for its laxative properties. It stimulates bowel movement and relieves constipation.

Directions: Add 5 g of sana makki powder to a glass of water. Drink before going to bed. Do this twice a month.

Avoid at all costs if you are a heart patient on medications like digoxin, warfarin or water pills (like many adults and most elderly people being treated for BP). This is because senna decreases potassium levels in the body.

Senna remains popular in traditional medicine and is often prescribed for constipation without considering potential medication interactions. I have included it on my list of home remedies because it's a first-choice laxative in the UK. However, it is not commonly given to aged patients. Remember that natural does *not* always mean safe! Herbal remedies like senna need to come with a clear warning about their interactions with BP and heart medications.

Diarrhoea

Traditionally, pomegranate peel has been used in China and Mexico to address diarrhoea, dysentery and stomach aches. Pomegranate seeds or juice can efficiently stop loose motions due to the fruit's anti-inflammatory effect on the gut. I would recommend making your own pomegranate peel powder for easy and effective consumption. Dry the pomegranate peels thoroughly in the sun or a grill set to a low temperature to avoid burning. Then use a dry grinder to create a fine powder.

Directions: Add one teaspoon of pomegranate peel powder to one cup of water. Boil and strain. Add honey and five drops of lemon juice before drinking. You can consume this beverage once or twice a day.

IBS-D

Indications: Stomach pain, bloating, diarrhoea

IBS-D, or irritable bowel syndrome with diarrhoea predominance, is a long-lasting digestive disorder that affects the large intestine. It's a complicated condition that greatly reduces quality of life, caused by several factors such as chemical abnormalities in the gut, a weak intestinal barrier, changes in gut bacteria, stress and genetics.

Like diarrhoea caused by factors other than IBS, pomegranate peel powder dissolved in warm water can help. It activates multiple mechanisms that restore intestinal barrier function and the secretory cells of the colon. The beneficial compounds present in pomegranate peel can modify cellular pathways and stop the inflammatory cell attack on the colon. However, while pomegranate peel powder may help with mild, non-infectious diarrhoea, it's not a substitute for medical treatment if symptoms are severe, persistent or due to infection.

Avoid for children under two years of age unless guided by a healthcare provider. Small, age-appropriate doses can help with mild diarrhoea in older children. For two- to five-year-olds, administer 1/8 to 1/4 teaspoon (about 0.25–0.5 g) once daily. For six- to twelve-year-olds, 1/4 to 1/2 teaspoon (about 0.5 g–1 g) once or twice daily. Mix the powder with a small amount of warm water or honey and serve after meals. Only appropriate for short-term use – no more than two to three days. Always consult a paediatrician beforehand, especially if the child has a fever, blood in their stool or signs of dehydration.

IBS-C

Indications: Abdominal ache, abdominal cramps, gripping sensation

IBS-C is a form of irritable bowel syndrome where constipation is the main symptom. People with IBS-C often experience infrequent bowel movements, hard or lumpy stools, abdominal pain and bloating. The pain usually reduces after passing stool. IBS-C is a functional gut disorder, meaning there's no visible damage to the digestive tract but the bowel doesn't work properly. It is influenced by factors like stress, gut-brain axis dysfunction, slow intestinal motility and altered gut bacteria.

Barley water is a great remedy to have on hand for those dealing with IBS-C – you can find the recipe in Chapter 10. Additionally, a coriander, cumin and fenugreek-based anti-dyspeptic can help curb accompanying symptoms like flatulence, bloating and appetite loss.

Directions: Take one tablespoon each of cumin (jeera) and fenugreek (methi) seeds, along with two tablespoons of coriander seeds. Grind the ingredients separately before combining them in a container. When you're ready to serve, brew one teaspoon (5 g) in 200 ml of boiling water. Drink the tea one hour before breakfast and dinner while warm.

Stomach ulcer

Indications: Acidity, heartburn, ulcers, indigestion

White pumpkin

Also known as ash gourd or winter melon.

Directions: Juice the pumpkin and drink this in the early morning. Consume regularly until symptoms reduce.

Avoid drinking this juice if you are pregnant. White pumpkin is generally considered safe during pregnancy when cooked and eaten as part of a balanced diet. However, the cooling and drying nature of its juice does not suit expectant mothers. It can cause excess urine production, low BP and electrolyte disturbance.

Gut inflammation and irritation

From ancient texts to laboratory studies, aloe vera has been reputed as a powerful healing plant. It bridges the wisdom of traditional medicine with the validation of modern science, offering holistic support for internal and external health. Known as *Kumari* in Ayurveda, it is valued for balancing Pitta and supporting liver health, stable menstruation and digestive cooling. Unani regards aloe (Sabir) as a potent detoxifier and liver stimulant, used to treat constipation, jaundice and inflammatory conditions. In TCM, aloe (Lu Hui) is part of formulations for liver detoxification, parasitic infections and heat-clearing therapies.

Aloe vera has a strong connection with gut wellness. Its gel contains mucopolysaccharides, which coat and soothe the gastrointestinal lining, thus aiding the management of gastritis, ulcers and IBS. Aloe's anti-inflammatory action helps reduce gut inflammation and irritation. It has prebiotic properties that support the growth of beneficial gut bacteria. It also accelerates the healing of gastric ulcers by increasing mucous production and improving microcirculation.

Aloe vera-based digestive

Blend two tablespoons of fresh aloe vera gel with one cup of water or coconut water. Add one teaspoon of honey and a few drops of lemon juice if desired. Drink this refreshing mix on an empty stomach in the morning, two to three times a week. It will help soothe the gut lining, ease acidity, improve digestion and relieve constipation naturally.

Night-time aloe vera tonic

Add two teaspoons of aloe vera gel to a cup of chamomile tea or warm water. Add a pinch of nutmeg powder, honey and optional pure rose water to taste. Drink thirty to sixty minutes before bedtime. This calming tonic soothes the stomach lining, relaxes the digestive tract and eases bloating and acidity. Nutmeg's gentle sedative effect can counteract mild insomnia while taking care of overnight digestion and gut repair. One course should last between ten to twelve days, with a gap of seven days between courses.

Avoid if pregnant! The yellow sap just beneath the aloe leaf's skin has strong laxative properties, which can trigger uterine contractions and even increase chances of miscarriage or premature labour. It may also cause electrolyte imbalance and diarrhoea, which are risky for pregnant people. Even if the latex is removed, avoid oral products like toothpastes that contain aloe during pregnancy due to limited human safety data.

Metabolic Diseases

Diabetes

Alternate and Western medicine agree that fenugreek or methi seed is an anti-diabetic agent. The seed's fibre content – galactomannan – helps lower blood sugar levels due to its ability to slow down carbohydrate absorption. Its chemical components aid the reversal of insulin resistance at the level of muscle and adipose tissue receptors. Even though most doctors acknowledge this effect of methi seeds, we don't know the right method or quantity to recommend. One of my colleagues was asked by a patient whether they should consume methi seeds dry or soaked. His lack of awareness led him to say it didn't matter. But matter it does.

Fenugreek seeds are high in soluble fibre, aiding digestion and regulating blood sugar, making them beneficial for diabetes and constipation. If you compare the nutritional content of dry versus soaked methi piecemeal, the former contains more fibre. Like sheep, we have been trained to follow the yellow brick road of 'more fibre, less calories'. But if there is anything I hope you have picked up from this book, it's that experiments in the lab cannot measure exactly how your body will respond to food – in particular, whole foods.

When soaked, methi seeds change from a hot food to a cooling food in some ways. This effect is more pronounced in Kapha-predominant individuals. Soaking methi seeds releases mucilage, though not as significantly as sabja seeds. This process reduces the 'heat' of methi seeds and the released mucilage has a soothing effect on the digestive tract. Additionally, soaking the seeds lessens their bitterness, making them easier on our taste buds. It also increases nutrient bioavailability, enhancing absorption in the body.

For Vata individuals, soaked fenugreek seeds can be particularly beneficial due to their hydrating and soothing properties. For Pitta individuals, fenugreek seeds should be consumed in moderation, preferably soaked to reduce their heating effect. For Kapha individuals, both dry and soaked fenugreek seeds are beneficial. However, dry seeds may be more effective for reducing excess Kapha due to their bitter and pungent properties. One of my patients with borderline diabetes ended up experiencing sinus congestion after regularly drinking methi water and eating soaked seeds. She had to resort to dry seeds and sprouted methi to benefit from this superfood minus the sniffles.

Directions: To control blood sugar levels, soak one to two tablespoons of methi seeds overnight. Drink this mixture in the morning – make sure to chew the seeds!

Avoid when pregnant because regular high intake can cause preterm labour.

Diabetic nephropathy

Indications: Swelling in the feet, ankles or hands, foamy urine, frequent night-time urination, fatigue, poor appetite, especially in advanced stages

When diabetes affects the kidneys, they become less efficient at filtering waste from blood. Barley water is a fail-safe way to improve kidney function in diabetes. It is a natural diuretic, blood sugar stabilizer and kidney protector, making it a gentle yet effective adjuvant remedy for diabetic nephropathy. Refer to Chapter 10 to make barley water at home and have one glass a day.

People who require dialysis often have very poor appetites. Despite the need for nourishing food, the toxin build-up caused by poor kidney function suppresses appetite and gives rise to terrible nausea. In such cases, patients can consume barley porridge or khichdi, even in little quantities. It is nutritious, supports kidney health and helps to excrete the toxin build-up.

Diabetic neuropathy

Indications: Tingling, numbness, burning, stabbing or shooting pain, muscle weakness, loss of balance

This is one of the most common complications of diabetes and can significantly affect daily movement and safety. High blood sugar damages nerves, especially in the feet and hands, leading to a whole host of inconvenient and painful symptoms.

Roghan-e-Badam (sweet almond oil)

Studies show that almond oil supports myelin sheath integrity and reduces demyelination – a key feature of diabetic neuropathy. The monounsaturated fatty acids (MUFAs) in almonds enhance nerve cell membrane fluidity and function. Sweet almond oil helps lower LDL cholesterol and triglycerides while improving insulin sensitivity, indirectly protecting against further nerve damage caused by uncontrolled blood glucose and poor circulation.[66] The healthy fats in almond oil may support microcirculation, which is often compromised in diabetic neuropathy. Better blood flow delivers nutrients and oxygen to the affected nerves more effectively, promoting healing and reducing numbness or burning sensations.

Directions: Consume one teaspoon (5 ml) of cold-pressed, food-grade sweet almond oil in the morning on an empty stomach. If you prefer, mix with warm milk. Doing so daily can help nourish the nerves and relieve tingling. Massaging the affected areas with the oil will also provide relief.

Mehendi

Mehendi or henna (*Lawsonia inermis*) has been used traditionally for its cooling, anti-inflammatory and antimicrobial effects. When applied topically, it helps ease burning, tingling and numbness in the hands and feet. Its cooling nature and mild vasodilation are thought to improve microcirculation to distal nerves while also calming local immune activity and reducing nerve irritation.

Animal studies suggest possible neuroprotective effects, though human data is limited.[67] Still, many find symptomatic relief. An aunt of mine with diabetic neuropathy applies henna to her soles every other day; the relief is temporary but significant. While not a cure, henna can serve as supportive care alongside blood sugar management.

Directions: Mix pure henna powder with water or rose water until it forms a smooth paste. Let it rest for a few hours. Clean and dry the feet or hands before applying a thin, even layer of the paste over the soles or palms, focusing on the most sensitive areas. Leave it on for twenty to sixty minutes (depending on comfort) and let it air-dry before rinsing with cool water. Repeat two to three times a week or as needed.

Avoid premixed commercial cones that may contain harmful additives. Always do a patch test first.

High blood pressure

The Sidr tree (*ber ka ped* in Hindi), known for its calming, anti-inflammatory and cardiotonic properties, is traditionally used in prophetic medicine. Its leaves and fruits contain flavonoids, saponins and alkaloids that may help relax blood vessels, reduce oxidative stress and lower BP, albeit mildly.
Directions: Boil five to seven dried ber leaves in one cup of water for five to seven minutes. Strain and drink once a day. Alternatively, have half a teaspoon of ber powder (made by pounding the leaf, not in a grinder) mixed with warm water or honey once daily.

Avoid drinking more than one cup a day as your BP might drastically reduce and cause a fainting spell. If you feel lightheaded, stop consuming the tea altogether and get your BP checked.

Adding pomegranate seeds or juice to your diet four or five times a week can also have a positive impact on BP. As always, do not overdo it – even whole foods can interfere with BP medication when in excess.

Liver

The liver quietly works day and night to filter toxins, balance blood sugar and process everything from meals to medicines to *madira*. Sometimes lifestyle factors like excess intake of alcohol, fatty foods or long-term medication use overwork it, leading to common issues such as fatty liver or mild inflammation. Gentle natural supports like aloe vera gel can help soothe and protect the liver to some extent. Still, it's important to remember that aloe will not reverse serious liver diseases like cirrhosis, hepatitis or cancer, where professional treatment is essential.

Directions: To make aloe vera gel at home, choose a mature, thick leaf from the *Aloe barbadensis miller* plant – the safe, edible variety. Wash the leaf thoroughly and cut off the base to let the yellow sap (aloin) drain for about twenty to thirty minutes. Aloin is a bitter laxative that should not be consumed. Once drained, trim the spiky edges, peel off the green skin and scoop out the clear gel inside. Blend the gel for a smooth texture and store it in a clean jar in the fridge for up to one week.

If you choose to use store-bought aloe, ensure that it is labelled food-grade or 100 per cent edible. Unlike cosmetic aloe products that are meant for external use, edible gel is clear with no added chemicals or fragrances.

To improve liver and gut health you can consume one teaspoon of aloe vera gel in the morning on an empty stomach.

Prostate and Urinary Health

BPH

The prostate is a gland found only in males, situated just below the bladder and surrounding the urethra. It is a crucial component of the male reproductive system, responsible for producing seminal fluid that nourishes and transports sperm during ejaculation.

As I explained in Chapter 8, the prostate enlarges with age due to a condition called benign prostatic hyperplasia (BPH). Symptoms include frequent urination, difficulty starting or maintaining a urine stream, weak urine flow, dribbling after urination and a feeling of incomplete bladder emptying.

Pumpkin seeds

Though tiny, pumpkin seeds have been recognized for their medicinal benefits for centuries. The phytochemicals in pumpkin seeds may reduce the effects of dihydrotestosterone – a powerful metabolite of testosterone that builds up in the prostate and causes it to grow. They may also block the conversion of testosterone into dihydrotestosterone. People experiencing pain in the abdomen, frequent urination and burning sensation while urinating stand to benefit from daily consumption of pumpkin seeds, too.

Directions: Consume one teaspoon of pumpkin seeds followed by a walnut before lunch and dinner daily.

Enuresis

Enuresis means involuntary urination, especially during sleep (nocturnal enuresis). While it is more common in children, older men with BPH may experience it as a symptom of advanced lower urinary tract dysfunction.

Black sesame

In TCM and Ayurveda, black sesame is considered nourishing for the kidneys and adrenals – organs linked to bladder and urine control. It addresses delayed bladder maturity in children. It is a safe intervention provided the child is not allergic to sesame.

Directions: A daily dose between 1/2 to one teaspoon of ground black sesame seeds is effective. Can be roasted or raw. Mix the powder with equal amounts of sugar (to make it more palatable) and feed it to the child an hour before bedtime. Remember to start small for young children and try mix-ins like honey, dates or warm milk.

Avoid for the day if your child's bedtime is less than an hour away. Hitting the bed immediately after consuming black sesame can lead to morning acidity and reflux. The seed has a hot nature, so overconsumption can lead to diarrhoea.

Olive oil massage

Olive oil contains oleic acid and squalene, which have mild anti-spasmodic and tissue-healing properties. A gentle abdominal massage encourages the body to relax (rest-and-digest response by the parasympathetic nerves), regulating bladder signalling and the night-time urination reflex.

Directions: Warm olive oil before rubbing it on the lower abdomen (below the belly button). Gently massage the oil in a circular fashion for five minutes. This can be done regularly after passing urine and before sleeping to reduce night-time urine urges and bedwetting.

Uric acid

Uric acid is a waste product formed when the body breaks down purines – substances found naturally in your cells and certain foods (e.g., red meat, seafood, alcohol). Normally, uric acid dissolves in the blood, passes through the kidneys and is excreted in urine. However, if the body produces too much or the kidneys excrete too little, uric acid build-up results in a condition called hyperuricemia.

When uric acid levels rise too high, it begins to form needle-like crystals in the spaces between joints. These trigger an intense immune response, causing pain, redness, swelling and heat. You've likely heard of gout – inflammatory arthritis caused by uric acid crystal deposition in joints, most commonly the big toe.

There are a couple of drugs which reduce uric acid levels or inflammatory activity but they come with a host of side effects. Though food therapy has a limited role in acute ongoing arthritis, it can work well for prevention. Black seeds (kalonji) improve renal clearance of uric acid by protecting and enhancing kidney function.

Directions: You will need four tablespoons (50 g) each of black, fenugreek and ajwain seeds. Mix only after grinding the ingredients separately. Store the seed mix in an airtight container. Consume one teaspoon (5 g) on an empty stomach as well as one hour after dinner. A course should last ten to fifteen days with a break of one week between courses.

Avoid black seed oil in high doses if on blood thinners or multiple heart medications. Always start with a low dose if you're on prescription meds. Monitor BP (if on BP medication), INR (if on the blood thinner warfarin) and blood sugar (fenugreek can cause a dip).

Gallbladder and Kidney

Gallstones

Gallstones are hardened deposits that form in the gallbladder. This happens when substances in bile like cholesterol, bile salts or bilirubin become imbalanced and crystallize. Modern medicine has a wait-and-watch policy for treating gallstones. Basically, we keep an eye on your annual ultrasound to monitor the growth of that precious stone. This approach totally disregards the time advantage offered by the slow formation of the stone and the usefulness of dietary therapy.

Middle-aged women are up to three times more likely to develop gallstones than men in the same stage of life.[68] This tendency has a lot to do with hormones: increased oestrogen and progesterone during pregnancy or fluctuations upon using birth control pills or hormone therapy for menopause. These hormones make the liver release more cholesterol into bile, slowing the emptying of the gallbladder. The bile sits for longer, making it easier for stones to form.

Black seeds (kalonji)

Kalonji has been traditionally used for liver and gallbladder health. It stimulates bile secretion, which may prevent bile stagnation – a key factor in gallstone formation. Thymoquinone, the main compound in black seed, lowers cholesterol levels in bile. The seed's antioxidants help protect the liver and bile ducts, improving overall bile quality. It also supports liver function, helping the organ process and balance bile components more efficiently.

Directions: Mix half a teaspoon of kalonji oil into hot water. Sweeten with honey and drink to dissolve gallstones. This home remedy can be consumed twice a day, in the morning and evening. Use consistently for four to six weeks but take a week-long break after every month of use.

Avoid if you have symptoms like severe upper abdominal pain, pain radiating to your back or shoulder, fever, vomiting or jaundice. Kalonji may prevent or slow the progression of gallstones but it is unlikely to dissolve stones that are large, calcified or have medical complications. Seek immediate medical attention and do not attempt to remedy the gallstones at home.

The olive oil-apple protocol

This is a simple home remedy taken from Western naturopathy that can help reverse gallstone formation. While this therapy does not 'dissolve' preexisting stones, it helps expel the deposits formed in the gallbladder by softening, mobilizing and flushing biliary sludge while reducing the digestive load on the liver–gallbladder axis. Apple's malic acid gently chelates calcium and loosens small, compact cholesterol stones, making them more pliable. Olive oil triggers a strong but smoother gallbladder emptying reflex, encouraging the expulsion of softened sludge and small stones.

The first step is to shift to a simple low-fat, plant-based (vegan) diet for a few days. This will temporarily minimize gallbladder contractions and bile thickening, giving the organ a 'rest phase' while improving bile fluidity through higher fibre intake and lower saturated fat. Keep in mind that this protocol is best understood as supportive and preventive - not a replacement for proper diagnosis or treatment when symptomatic gallstones are present.

Directions: Consume two teaspoons of olive oil dissolved in a glass of warm water in the morning. Follow this with a twenty-minute walk. For the first seven days of this therapy, eat an apple a day. Take a week's break after a two-week course.

Apple cider vinegar (ACV)

The recent trend of mindlessly chugging ACV on an empty stomach has made me a somewhat reluctant rider in the apple cider vinegar bandwagon. However, vinegar is the best condiment ever according to prophetic medicine and modern science confirms this view. ACV reduces stone progression and improves gallbladder volume and wall thickness. It also enhances digestion by boosting gut movement and the release of a hormone called cholecystokinin. This hormone makes the gallbladder contract and opens the bile duct, which helps push out small gallstones.

Directions: Combine one teaspoon of ACV with 200 ml (around one glass) of water. Add one teaspoon each of grapefruit/orange juice and lemon juice. Consume this mixture twice a day, one hour before breakfast and dinner. This course can be continued for a month. For the first seven days, eat an apple every morning. Take a two-week break before starting the next course.

Avoid for ulcer patients.

Kidney stones

Kidney stones are hard deposits that are formed when urine becomes overly concentrated. Minerals such as calcium, oxalate and uric acid crystallize and stick together, forming stones of varying sizes. These stones may stay in the kidney or travel down the urinary tract, often causing sharp, intense pain, blood in the urine, nausea, vomiting and difficulty urinating.

Treatment depends on the size and type of stone. Smaller stones often pass naturally with increased fluid intake and pain management. However, larger or obstructive stones may require medical or surgical procedures.

Natural management plays a key role in reducing recurrence. Staying well-hydrated is essential to prevent urine concentration and stone formation. Avoiding oxalate-rich foods (e.g., spinach, salt, animal protein) can help. Citrate-rich foods like lemons and oranges may inhibit stone formation. Try herbal remedies such as black seed and barley water (recipes above) to support kidney function, dissolve small stones and promote smoother urine flow. Other food therapies for kidney stones include banana stem juice in the early morning and carrot-radish juice once a day.

Skincare

Moles

When I was twelve years old, I developed a mole on my cheek. It should have been considered a beauty spot but alas, I had brothers. They teased me endlessly – that the mole would grow in size, that tiny hairs would sprout from it. These were the same brothers who told me I was found in the garbage bin as a baby, so you get the drift!

Back then, a neighbour told my mom that the mole would fade if I applied kalonji paste on it. And fade it did – in just one week!

Directions: To make kalonji paste, pound black seeds along with a little water. The powder need not be too fine. The paste isn't like a typical face pack; it is gritty and sticks rather than spreads. Apply it on the skin with your fingertips - gently, no rubbing! Leave it on for ten minutes and wash off with warm water.

Active acne and scarring

In my thirties my skin developed a fresh crop of acne as if I'd just hit puberty. Despite my best efforts to not pick and poke the pimples, I got a fresh crop of acne marks to match. I waited in vain for the stubborn pink marks to subside but they didn't. That is until I remembered the kalonji paste that had tackled my mole.

Directions: If you're experiencing active acne, consume five to ten kalonji seeds daily with water on an empty stomach. In case of acne scarring, apply kalonji paste on the affected area.

Kalonji can also help manage conditions like psoriasis, dermatitis and hives. However, these conditions require longstanding treatment and there hasn't been enough research into the interaction of kalonji with topical drugs. Until we get more data, you can safely consume five to ten seeds of kalonji with water on an empty stomach every morning for all kinds of skin issues.

13

FOODS FOR THE FEMININE LIFECYCLE

The resilience and adaptability of women transcends time and circumstance. If men have brute strength, women have tolerance and tenacity. Whether navigating complexities of family life, pursuing professional goals, challenging societal norms or confronting personal struggles, women exhibit an innate ability to adapt, evolve and thrive. This resilience is not merely a response to external pressures but a reflection of their indomitable spirit. But one cannot pour from an empty cup. We need to keep refilling our cups with nourishment – the ultimate form of self-care.

Menstruation

The liver plays a vital role in regulating hormones, especially those involved in the menstrual cycle. It breaks down and detoxifies the likes of oestrogen, progesterone and testosterone. When the liver is stressed due to fat, iron or scar tissue build-up in its filtering channels (sinusoids) – such as in fatty liver – this process is disrupted.

Oestrogen, when not cleared properly, may cause heavy periods, PMS or conditions like endometriosis due to a state of oestrogen dominance. Similarly, poor progesterone metabolism can lead to low progesterone levels, resulting in irregular cycles, short luteal phases or fertility issues. Even testosterone, if not broken down properly, can accumulate and contribute to problems like acne, irregular periods or PCOS. In severe cases, impaired liver detoxification leads to overall hormonal imbalances and inflammation. This affects not just menstrual health but also broader hormonal regulation. Keeping the liver healthy by maintaining a clean diet, ample hydration and managing toxins supports smoother hormone metabolism and a more balanced menstrual cycle.

Period-related diarrhoea and cramps (dysmenorrhea) are both linked to hormone-like compounds called prostaglandins. During menstruation, the endometrial lining of the uterus releases high levels of prostaglandins, especially in the first few days of a period. Prostaglandins stimulate the smooth muscles of the uterus, causing it to contract. These contractions help shed the uterine lining but can also be painful, especially if the uterus contracts intensely or if blood flow is temporarily restricted to the uterine muscles.

Prostaglandins also affect other smooth muscles, such as those in the digestive tract. This can lead to increased bowel contractions, resulting in loose stools. This mechanism explains why period cramps and diarrhoea often occur in conjunction and why they tend to be most intense at the start of menstruation when prostaglandin levels are highest.

Period cramps

Applying lavender essential oil to the lower abdomen during menstruation can help relieve cramps and discomfort. Its main active compounds have a natural antispasmodic effect, easing the painful contractions of the uterus. Lavender also reduces inflammation by lowering prostaglandin levels. It relieves pain by calming nerve activity and modulating pain signals. When applied topically or inhaled, lavender oil helps relax the nervous system, control cortisol levels and promote a sense of calm, countering the physical and emotional symptoms of menstruation.

To use, dilute two to three drops of lavender essential oil in coconut or sesame oil and gently massage the lower abdomen with circular motions. This can be done once or twice a day during menstruation. PMS symptoms can also be treated with lavender oil when it is diluted and applied behind the ears. This has a calming effect on the mind and enables more restful sleep.

Lavender's soothing properties make it a safe and effective natural remedy for managing period pain, especially when combined with rest, heat therapy and deep breathing. Additionally, you can sip on ginger or cinnamon tea to help relieve cramps.

Period bloating

Like cramping and diarrhoea, prostaglandin excess during periods can result in bloating. To temper this, avoid cold and raw foods in favour of warm, nourishing meals. An exception to this is eating raw bananas, as they can help with controlling diarrhoea.

Saunf (fennel seed) has muscle-relaxant properties and works as an antispasmodic. It reduces the formation of gas bubbles and promotes the expulsion of excess gas, alleviating uncomfortable bloating. Chew the seeds to relieve cramps and bloating or opt for cumin-fennel tea to get rid of the bloat and diarrhoea. Brew one teaspoon each of cumin and fennel in hot water. Sip while warm.

Spotting before periods

Although multifactorial, spotting before periods can be considered a disorder due to uterine weakness or liver dysfunction. In traditional medicine, spotting is thought to be caused by an overdrive of body heat. Try the following home remedies:

- **Fig-based nabeez** – Soak two to three figs overnight; eat on an empty stomach. Improves digestion and uterine tone.
- **Rose water and honey** – Add one teaspoon of each to warm water; drink at night. Mild uterine tonic, balances heat.

Irregular cycles

Unlike spotting, irregular periods are considered a result of cold temperament, uterine weakness or stress.

- **Sesame seeds and jaggery** – One teaspoon each, crushed, taken during the luteal phase. The second half of your menstrual cycle, it starts around day fifteen in a typical twenty-eight-day cycle and lasts until your period begins. During this phase, the uterine lining thickens to prepare for a possible pregnancy. The sesame-jaggery combo is warming in nature and stimulates menstruation, skipping the spotting.
- **Ajwain tea** – Brew half a teaspoon of ajwain in boiling water. Drink before breakfast for ten days. Enhances uterine blood flow.
- **Aloe vera gel** – Have one to two teaspoons of fresh aloe vera gel mixed with honey or jaggery on an empty stomach before breakfast. You can start this course any day after your period ends. Continue for ten to fifteen days, leading up to your next expected period. Repeat monthly until your cycle regularizes. This usually takes two to three months.
- **Aloe vera juice** (unsweetened) – Drink 10–20 ml diluted with water daily for ten to fifteen days before your expected period. Do not use during active menstruation if you have heavy flow, as aloe has a mild uterine stimulating effect.

PCOS

Excess androgens due to liver sluggishness in PCOS may give rise to unwanted facial and body hair. You can try:

- **Mint and cinnamon tea** – One cup a day. Balances hormones and reduces androgenic symptoms.
- **Powdered fenugreek seeds** – 1/4 teaspoon with honey daily. Supports endocrine balance.

Heavy bleeding

Coriander seeds provide a variety of benefits. They act as a gentle liver tonic and have cooling, anti-inflammatory, antioxidant and stress-reducing properties that help calm the body and support overall balance. Together, these actions make coriander a valuable remedy for managing conditions linked to excess body heat including skin irritation, menstrual imbalances and digestive discomfort. Thus, a cold infusion of coriander seeds is a great addition to your diet if you're experiencing heavy bleeding. Soak one teaspoon of seeds in water overnight. Strain and drink the next morning.

You can also have half a teaspoon of pomegranate peel powder with honey twice a day. This paste works as an astringent and has a cooling effect on the body.

Infections

Be it the persistent urinary infection or the itching-of-nightmares yeast infection, the first step is to not be tempted to overclean down below. This strips away the natural protective oils and good bacteria that keep the vaginal and vulval microbiome in balance. The resulting dryness and micro-tears only intensify the burning and itching, creating a cycle that keeps worsening the more you try to 'clean'. Frequent washing also disrupts the acidic pH that stops yeast and harmful bacteria from multiplying. Before you are tempted to reach for a pill, here are some home remedies to please the pee.

Vaginal yeast infection

1. **Barley**: Soothes internal inflammation, reduces excess moisture and supports urinary and vaginal tract cleansing. Barley water or soup can be consumed daily.
2. **Pomegranate:** Antifungal and astringent; helps reduce discharge and soothes mucosal membranes. Eat fresh pomegranate or drink diluted pomegranate juice.

Urinary tract infection

Urinary tract infections are hell-sent. Your hoo-hoo is on fire and the toilet beckons every few minutes. The frequent urine pressure and trickle of urine are agony in its purest form. UTIs are caused by bacteria, most often *E. coli*, entering and multiplying in the urinary tract. It typically leads to symptoms like burning urine, frequent urge to urinate, discomfort and cloudy or strong-smelling urine. Many people recommend cranberry juice to relieve the burning. But the Tetra Pak versions are loaded with added sugars – which can actually feed harmful bacteria – and may lack sufficient active compounds like proanthocyanidins, making them far less effective than fresh, unsweetened cranberry extract or concentrate. Even if you find cranberry extract or capsules, be cautious, as they can cause digestive discomfort, increase kidney-stone risk or interact with certain medications if consumed in excess. So, be careful before you recommend it to your mum.

Here is a rundown of safer alternatives which will give cranberry a run for its money.

1. **Barley water**: Acts as a mild diuretic, soothes inflamed urinary tract, flushes out infection. Sip throughout the day.
2. **Cucumber**: Hydrating, diuretic and cooling; reduces burning during urination. Eat raw or juice and drink with a pinch of salt.
3. **Sugarcane juice**: Hydrating, supports urinary tract mucosal integrity and urine flow, relieves burning sensation. Drink fresh juice in moderation. Diabetics should not exceed one glass a day.
4. **Coriander seed water**: Mild diuretic, supports biofilm formation, prevents recurrence. Soak one tablespoon of crushed seeds overnight in water. Strain and drink in the morning.

Pregnancy

Pregnancy is a deeply challenging and transformative time in a woman's life. The Quran refers to it as 'weakness upon weakness', acknowledging the physical and emotional demands experienced by expecting mothers.[69] In Islamic tradition, mothers are held in the highest regard. This is reflected in the well-known saying, 'Paradise lies at the feet of the mother.'

Eating during pregnancy

According to Ayurveda, certain foods should be avoided during pregnancy as they tend to aggravate Pitta (heat) and Vata (dryness) in the body to the point of imbalance. These include spicy, sour, fried and oily foods such as pickles and other fermented products. Limit their consumption to maintain a calm and balanced internal environment during pregnancy.

Instead, prioritize warm, cooked and easily digestible foods that support both the mother and developing baby. Examples include khichdi, soups and cooked vegetables – all gentle on the digestive system. Include nourishing items like ghee and warm milk flavoured with mild spices such as cardamom. These help provide essential nutrients and promote balance. Sweet and wholesome fruits like mangoes, figs, dates, bananas, pomegranates and cooked apples are also encouraged for their nourishing qualities. Herbal teas made from ginger or cumin are commonly recommended, as they help soothe the digestive tract and prevent discomfort.

In the first trimester, focus on light, easy-to-digest meals. In the third, choose foods that strengthen and tone the uterus like dates, warm milk, ghee and saffron. Pregnancy is not the time to go crazy experimenting with unfamiliar foods or the next fad diet. The body needs to be nourished without straining to digest raw or unfamiliar foods. However, there is one method to whip out simple meals, reduce glucose spikes and keep yourself full for longer that I would recommend you try even if it is unfamiliar. That is the humble practice of *roti choorna*.

Soupy meals enhance satiety and slow down digestion by preventing a phenomenon known as gastric sieving. This is a process whereby the liquid part of a meal leaves the stomach faster than the solid part, especially when the two are consumed separately. This can lead to quicker gastric emptying, reduced fullness and increased cravings.

When food and liquid are blended into a uniform mixture, this sieving is minimized. A study showed that only about a quarter of a mixed meal was emptied from the stomach thirty-five minutes after eating. The percentage was much higher when the solid and liquid components of a meal were consumed separately. This suggests that blended or soup-like meals slow digestion, keeping the stomach fuller for longer.

In traditional Indian diets, meals like choori roti with runny dal or paratha with paaya soup naturally adopt this principle, offering more stable energy levels. Such meal structures not only reduce overeating and snacking but also improve nutrient absorption by allowing more time for digestive action. Incorporating soupy meals is a simple and effective way to enhance satiety and support metabolic health, particularly for diabetic expectant mothers.

Managing pregnancy symptoms

Pregnant people can experience everything from fatigue and morning sickness to mood swings, increased urination and heartburn. These pesky symptoms can make pregnancy feel like a full-time job with zero breaks. Honestly, it is. Growing a bean into a human being ain't easy work. Thankfully, there are some homemade remedies that might give you a breather along the way.

1. **Morning sickness** – should be called all-day-long sickness! Nausea doesn't wait for the morning to hit.
    - **Ginger**: Boil fresh ginger slices in water and sip slowly.
    - **Pomegranate juice**: Fresh juice stabilizes digestion and reduces nausea.
    - **Cardamom (elaichi)**: Suck on cardamom seeds or drink warm cardamom-infused water.
    - **Jeera water**: Boil one teaspoon of cumin seeds in 1 litre of water, cool and sip throughout the day to reduce vomiting tendency.

2. **Acidity or heartburn**
    - **Cold milk with a pinch of cardamom**: A natural antacid.
    - **Saunf**: Chew after meals.
    - **Amla**: One teaspoon amla juice with honey in the morning.

- **Gulkand:** An excellent digestive aid when eaten after meals.
- **Hing:** Just a pinch in tadkas can aid digestion and reduce bloating, especially when cooking lentils or heavy foods.

3. **Constipation**
   - **Ghee with warm milk**: One teaspoon ghee in warm milk before bed.
   - **Nabeez:** Consume first thing in morning. Avoid in case of pregnancy-induced diabetes.

4. **Weakness** caused by increased metabolic demand or hormonal shifts. (For weakness due to low haemoglobin refer the section on anaemia).
   - **Dates with ghee**: Two soaked dates with a teaspoon of ghee or almond milk.
   - **Almonds**: Soaked and peeled almonds in the morning increase vitality.

5. **Backache or body aches**
   - **Warm sesame oil massage (Abhyanga):** Daily gentle massage.
   - **Turmeric milk**: Warm milk with 1/4 teaspoon turmeric at night for joint relief.

6. **Bloating, gas and constipation**
   - Hing (asafoetida) in coconut oil helps reduce dryness, itching, bloating, gas and mild constipation. Its resins and volatile oils stimulate local circulation, produce a gentle warming

effect, act on nerve endings to relieve cramps and improve gut transit. Mix 1/2 teaspoon of hing into a small amount of coconut oil and massage gently onto the abdomen.

7. **Swollen feet**
    - **Coriander seed tea**: Soak one teaspoon of seeds in water. Boil, cool and drink.
    - **Barley water**: Natural diuretic that reduces swelling.
    - **Foot elevation**: Rest feet on a pillow while sleeping to redirect blood circulation.

8. **Mood swings or anxiety**
    - **Milk with nutmeg and saffron:** 1/2 pinch each in warm milk. Soothing night drink.

9. **Burning urine or white vaginal discharge**
    - UTIs are common during pregnancy, so your doctor is likely to prescribe a urine routine test. For both urine infections and white discharge, drinking barley water will help ease the discomfort while flushing out pathogens. In addition, it reduces water retention.

Anaemia

Low haemoglobin causes weakness, fatigue, dull-looking eyes, shortness of breath on exertion and palpitations.

- **Date-based nabeez**: Have one hour after breakfast. Diabetics should steer clear.

- **Beetroot-carrot-apple juice**: Strain if desired or consume as a smoothie to retain fibre. Add pudina or lemon juice to taste and drink every morning.

Both remedies can help with anaemia regardless of cause. I also recommend them to patients experiencing heavy menstrual blood loss.

Post-Partum Health

During pregnancy, the mother's immune system undergoes changes to tolerate the developing foetus. Why tolerate? That's because the baby contains foreign genetic material. The shift towards a more tolerant immune response is required to prevent the body from rejecting the embryo. This shows up as low immunity in the mother, making her more susceptible to infections. Her body is willing to bend over backwards and then some to preserve her precious child.

After childbirth, the suppressed immune system can rebound sharply – a condition called Immune Reactivation Syndrome. This overactive response increases the mother's risk of infection and immune-related issues. Rest, nutrition and reduced exposure to potential pathogens can help mothers navigate this period of immune transition. This includes focusing on recovery and breastfeeding the baby, observing the six-week confinement period in the comfort of home and eating nourishing native foods

Your doshas post-partum

In Ayurveda, the post-partum period – also known as *Sutika Kala* – is a time of doshic chaos. Think of childbirth as a massive overhaul of both your organ systems and exterior environment.

Childbirth disproportionately increases downward Vata, which shows up as anxiety, insomnia, gas, bloating, constipation, joint pain and a general sense of instability. Let's take a closer look at how this imbalance takes shape in the post-partum body.

The biomechanics and biophysics of labour involve intense muscular, hormonal and pressure-related changes that can temporarily disrupt the normal evacuation functions. During labour, intra-abdominal pressure increases dramatically, which can weaken the pelvic floor. This can cause organs like the rectum, bladder and uterus to prolapse or be displaced, disturbing urination and defecation. The excess pressure can also cause nerve compression (e.g., of the pudendal nerve), impairing sensory and motor control of evacuation functions. Additionally, stretching of the connective tissues and ligaments supporting these organs may lead to temporary dysfunction.

Labour affects the autonomic nervous system, responsible for regulating muscle contractions in the intestines and urinary tract. The intense strain inhibits gut motility, causing constipation, bloating and urinary retention. Labour is hormonally driven, with surges of oxytocin, prostaglandins and endorphins. Oxytocin, while helping uterine contractions, temporarily inhibits bowel and bladder function. Excess prostaglandins can cause cramps or diarrhoea. But the opposite effects – constipation and gas retention – are more common. The excess hormones exhaust receptor sensitivity post-delivery, leading to sluggishness of the gut and bladder.

On the other hand, Pitta imbalance post-partum may manifest as irritability, anger, excessive sweating, acidity, skin rashes and inflammation. As a predominantly Pitta person, I experienced more of a Pitta imbalance during and after my pregnancies. I developed a breast abscess linked to mastitis and a thigh abscess. This book has been sitting on the back burner of my head ever since my through-and-through OBG commented, 'Why does this girl have so much Pitta?' And here I am nine years later, trying to puzzle through what my guru accidentally introduced me to.

While less common, post-partum Kapha imbalance is possible. This may happen if there is a tendency towards excessive weight gain, water retention or sluggish digestion.

Relief from breast engorgement and mastitis

Engorgement is the painful swelling of the breasts that occurs in the first two weeks after birth due to a sudden increase in milk volume, vascular congestion and fluid retention. This makes it difficult for the baby to latch onto the breast properly. If unmanaged, it can reduce milk supply and lead to complications like mastitis or infection. Excessive milk and engorgement may be a result of the baby drinking formula supplements (leading to inadequate drainage of breastmilk) or the mother receiving supplements to increase milk supply in the initial days.

The Ancient Greeks regularly used cabbage to relieve inflammation of the eye. Applying the same principle, the cold effect of cabbage can help reduce breast engorgement in new mothers.

Directions:

1. Peel the outside layer of the cabbage and use the inner leaves. Remove their veins and separate the leaves.
2. Apply the cabbage leaf to your breast, sparing the nipple. You can place it in the refrigerator for some time first to give prompt relief.
3. Once the leaf feels wilted – or after twenty minutes have passed – discard it.
4. The cabbage leaf can leave a distinct taste on your breast. Wash it off with water afterwards.

Avoid using this method more than thrice a day. The same mechanism that will soothe engorgement can reduce your milk supply, too! If you plan on weaning the baby, you can use cabbage leaf more often to reduce your milk supply naturally.

If you have any symptoms of a bacterial infection, immediately see your doctor. This could be fever with shivering, thinning of breast skin or collection of pus in your breast. The humble cabbage leaf might be able to counter inflammation but it is in no way strong enough to fight off a bacterial infection. Do not ignore these warning signs!

This raises the question: can new moms eat cabbage to reduce engorgement? The answer is a hard no. As I mentioned in Chapter 9, cabbage causes gassiness because of the carbohydrate raffinose and this effect can be passed on to the baby. To prevent this, it is better to steer clear of the cabbage family – including kale – post delivery.

After around two months, you can start eating this nutritious vegetable family again – in moderation and well-cooked (no coleslaw yet). I speak of moderation because that's about the time when women start hating the weighing scale and think of dieting. The cabbage juice diet detox is high up on the list of fad diets, so be wary!

The postpartum diet

Food should be cooked well and served warm. Stay clear of raw foods in this delicate phase of life.

Panchphoran

To ease digestive issues, reach for the panchphoran digestive – equal parts ajwain and methi seeds, saunf and kalonji. Take one teaspoon after meals. Ajwain relieves gas, methi supports metabolism, fennel enhances milk production and kalonji boosts immunity. A true multi-purpose remedy.

Panjeri

Another traditional and nourishing post-partum preparation is panjeri, a dry powdered snack made from dates, jaggery and dry fruits. It bolsters energy, lactation and recovery from childbirth.

Directions: Heat two tablespoons of ghee, add a cup of whole wheat flour and roast on low heat until the mixture turns golden-brown with a nutty aroma. Set aside to cool while you lightly roast two to three tablespoons of crushed dry fruits like almonds, cashews and walnuts. Remove the nuts and, in the same pan, fry cut, deseeded dates in ghee. Stir in one tablespoon of gond (edible gum) and cook until it puffs up. Combine all the ingredients, along with half a cup of powdered jaggery. Store in an airtight container. Every day you can enjoy a small portion by soaking it in warm milk.

Laddoos

Gond laddoos, made with ghee and gond, are especially beneficial. Both ingredients provide SCFAs that improve metabolism and help the body redistribute fat after pregnancy. Gond is also helpful for women recovering from gestational diabetes as it helps lower fasting glucose and promotes gradual, healthy weight loss.

Methi laddoos are excellent galactagogues – foods that enhance breast milk production – thanks to the lactation-supportive properties of fenugreek.

Poppy seed milk

Khus khus (poppy seed) milk soothes the nervous system, promotes better sleep and supports tissue repair during the post-partum phase.

Directions: Soak two teaspoons of khus khus and six almonds overnight. In the morning, grind them into a fine paste. Roast the paste in a teaspoon of ghee, then add a pinch of black pepper, cardamom and optionally saffron. Mix two to three teaspoons of this mixture into 300 ml of hot milk, sweeten to taste and enjoy for a calming, restorative sleep.

Halim

This comforting drink is an excellent source of calcium, iron and folic acid, so drink up. Soak halim (garden cress) seeds overnight in water. Boil along with some jaggery and ghee. Serve hot before breakfast. Filling and a great source of minerals, you can continue drinking this for as long as you like.

Non-vegetarian options

For non-vegetarians, bone soup – particularly paaya or *siraa* (goat head) soup – works wonders for counteracting the mineral depletion caused by breastfeeding. Serving bone broth with choori roti boosts nutrient absorption and satiety. The minerals present in the soup (gelatin, chondroitin, glucosamine) help restore the mother's digestive tract and bones. Rich in natural collagen and protein, broth supports skin plumpness and healing after delivery. Proline aids skin repair while its fellow amino acids calm the mind, balance hormones and promote restful sleep for the new mother.

EPILOGUE: THE RECLAIMED HUMAN

Researching this book has been a revelation. As an allopathic practitioner, I have spent years immersed in modern science. Yet this journey opened my eyes to the depth and nuance of traditional medicine – be it Unani, Ayurveda or TCM.

Though my book might have turned out to be an ode to Ayurvedic doshas, I do not claim that Ayurveda is the ultimate authority in medicine. It naturally ended up at the forefront of this work due to its accessible, in-depth concepts and my own foundational knowledge in this field. That said, the Unani theory of zaika had a profound impact on my research too. The subtle yet powerful connection between the taste of food and its bio-temperament – bridging our body's senses and responses – was a crucial piece of the puzzle.

This book was written to empower you to understand your temperament while cutting through the half-baked, fear-driven 'truths' often propagated by influencers and self-styled health gurus. I do not advocate replacing allopathy entirely – no single system of medicine is absolute. Instead, my goal was to expand on the so-called lifestyle modifications often mentioned in allopathic prescriptions and offer practical, holistic tools for everyday health.

Modern medicine has enabled remarkable research, discoveries and treatments. These cannot be dismissed entirely as trivial or corrupt, despite the looming presence of conflicts of interest in research and funding. To burn this legacy would make us no different than early medical 'reformers' like Rockefeller, Carnegie and Flexner, who reduced the curricula of hundreds of medical colleges to pure quackery overnight. That drastic disruption of traditional healing systems - driven by power and money - is one reason why we live in an era of unprecedented chronic disease despite medical advancements.

The most glaring drawback of modern medicine is its focus on addressing the consequences rather than root causes of disease. Authorities like WHO have sneakily shifted the focus from healing and cures to treatment and maintenance. While pragmatic, this principle is precisely what prevents modern medicine from achieving true holism. We cannot afford to keep pouring resources into managing symptoms while ignoring the larger picture. We are not merely the sum of our bodily functions. Health is a living, breathing symphony; a dynamic web of feedback loops and modulatory mechanisms, all influenced by temperament, environment and lifestyle.

A few words of caution are necessary. While this book emphasizes the power of time-tested remedies and lifestyle changes to restore balance, acute conditions demand the precision and urgency of modern medicine. Life-threatening illnesses such as cancer, severe infections or critical emergencies require conventional treatment. To ignore this reality would be reckless. Home remedies can support, complement and strengthen. But they must walk alongside – not instead of – the life-saving advances of modern medicine.

My vision is to bridge traditional wisdom with modern science – I do not intend to destroy either side of this bridge. Ultimately, this book would not exist without my medical training and grounding in science. These tools have allowed me to understand how tradition and modernity intersect; to honour the sagacity of the past while embracing present-day rigour. My earnest hope is that the insights in this book will eventually enrich mainstream medical education – embracing both scientific reductionism and traditional holism. A future where medicine is not a choice between two worlds but a union. Where healthcare is thoughtful, integrative and truly human.

ACKNOWLEDGEMENTS

This book lived in my mind for nearly a decade before I sat down to write it. The very first seed was planted by my husband. One day I was telling him that two of my patients had come in with the same 'heat-y' symptoms. He looked me straight in the eye and said, 'Just because modern medicine hasn't caught up doesn't mean they're wrong. Maybe you should think about it.' That moment stayed with me.

After the publication of my first book, *Newborns and New Moms*, and the busy year that followed, I finally returned to this idea that had been sitting on the back burner for so long. I am grateful to my agent, Anish, who embraced this book with so much enthusiasm. My heartfelt thanks to my brother Farooq, for his support through my book journey. I am also deeply appreciative of Kunal Bahl, co-founder of Snapdeal, and Ambi uncle for so generously endorsing my work. A big thanks to my editors Priyanka, Pujitha and Shreyoshee for their meticulous work and thoughtful suggestions that helped refine this manuscript.

My understanding of holistic traditions has been shaped by two practitioners. I owe special thanks to Ustad Abdul Ahad, who introduced me to Unani principles, TCM basics and food therapy. His classes helped me see the innate nature of food through the lens of taste – a perspective that opened many conceptual pathways for this book. I met Beth (@indigoforest.co), a midwife and holistic medicine practitioner, on Instagram. This chance meeting turned out to be a real game changer. Her recommendations from

Western naturopathy resources were invaluable for shaping my functional interpretation of the doshas.

Heartfelt thanks to my co-sister Nazia, for her steady encouragement and holding me accountable during spells of laziness and waning motivation. I am also grateful to Sayequa *bhabhi* for reviewing my early drafts and offering thoughtful, constructive feedback. My colleague and friend Dr Pradeep Kumar has been an invaluable intellectual companion and constant sounding board. Our endless discussions – about patient diets, clinical patterns, the intersections of traditional and modern medicine – sharpened many of the ideas explored in this book.

Lastly, I wish to acknowledge my children, who became editors of this book without being hired, enthusiastic reviewers of every revision without being asked and cover designers without being called upon. They read my drafts with a seriousness far beyond their years, jumped into revisions as though it were a grand adventure and took immense joy in imagining what the cover should look like. I will always treasure the folder of their wonderfully creative designs (though they never made it to the final stage) – each one reflecting their excitement, generosity and wholehearted participation in this journey.

NOTES

1. National Sponsors, Official website, American Diabetes Association. Available at: https://diabetes.org/about-us/supporting-partners/national-sponsors.
2. 'Healthier Smiles Community Service Grants', Official website, ADA Dental Health Foundation. Available at: https://adadhf.org.au/scholarships-and-grants/healthier-smiles-community-service-grants.
3. Marion Nestle, 'Oh, the Irony: Alcohol Companies Support Cancer Research', *The Atlantic*, 7 October 2010. Available at: https://www.theatlantic.com/health/archive/2010/10/oh-the-irony-alcohol-companies-support-cancer-research/64149/.
4. Official website, Breast Cancer Research Foundation. Available at: https://www.bcrf.org/majordonors.
5. Guadalupe Guzmán-Caroa, Fernando J. García López and Miguel Ángel Royo-Bordonada, 'Conflicts of interest among scientific foundations and societies in the field of childhood nutrition', *Gaceta Sanitaria*, Vol. 35(4), 2021, pp. 320–325. Available at: https://www.gacetasanitaria.org/en-conflicts-interest-among-scientific-foundations-articulo-S0213911120301278.
6. E. W. Dumbili, J. Bwalya and A. Osborne, 'Commercial determinants of infant and child health: A focus on Nestlé's baby food products marketed in Africa', *Ethics, Medicine and Public Health*, Vol. 33, 2025. Available at: https://www.sciencedirect.com/science/article/pii/S2352552525001458.
7. Jacqui Thornton, 'Nestlé accused of double standards over added sugar in baby products sold in poorer countries', *BMJ*, 18 April 2024. Available at: https://www.bmj.com/content/385/bmj.q898.
8. Aylin Elci, 'What is the sugar scandal hitting Nestlé and what happens now?', *Euronews*, 19 April 2024. Available at: https://www.euronews.com/health/2024/04/19/what-is-the-sugar-scandal-hitting-nestle-and-what-happens-now.
9. Robert Lustig, *Metabolical* (New York: HarperCollins, 2021).
10. 'Tobacco money and medical research' (Editorial), *Nature Medicine*, Vol. 5, 1999, p. 125. Available at: https://www.nature.com/articles/nm0299_125.
11. Sreelakshmi Nair, 'Quinoa Cultivation: Economic plight of Bolivian farmers', Economics Declassified, 9 December 2022. Available at: https://economicsdeclassified.wordpress.com/2022/12/09/quinoa-cultivation-economic-plight-of-bolivian-farmers/.

12. Denisse Román-Burgos and Ricardo F. Macip-Ríos, 'Export quality: the historical bloc, state of exception, and the hegemonic process in the avocado enclave of Michoacán', *Dialectical Anthropology*, Vol. 46, 2022, pp. 225–246. Available at: https://link.springer.com/article/10.1007/s10624-022-09662-9?.
13. Dayeeta Das, 'Avocado Boom Comes At A Price In Portugal's Parched Algarve', *European Supermarket Magazine*, 13 October 2020. Available at: https://www.esmmagazine.com/fresh-produce/avocado-boom-comes-at-a-price-in-portugals-parched-algarve-111292.
14. 'Popular avocado cultivation is starting to take its toll in southern Portugal' (Editorial), Tridge, 15 October 2020. Available at: https://www.tridge.com/news/popular-avocado-cultivation-is-starting-to-take-it/.
15. George Dunea, 'Spinach: The great myth', *Hektoen International*, Vol. 14(4), 2022. Available at: https://hekint.org/2022/07/18/spinach-the-great-myth/.
16. Michael K. McMullen, Julie M. Whitehouse and Anthony Towell, 'Bitters: Time for a New Paradigm', *Evidence-Based Complementary and Alternative Medicine*, 2015. Available at: https://www.ncbi.nlm.nih.gov/pmc/articles/PMC4446506/.
17. Ibid.
18. Hannah E. R. Frank, et al., 'The evolution of sour taste', *Proceedings of the Royal Society B*, Vol. 289, 2022. Available at: https://pubmed.ncbi.nlm.nih.gov/35135352/.
19. Ibid.
20. Jasmin Khateeb, Eyal Fuchs and Mogher Khamaisi, 'Diabetes and Lung Disease: An Underestimated Relationship', *Review of Diabetic Studies*, Vol. 15, 2019, pp. 1–15. Available at: https://pmc.ncbi.nlm.nih.gov/articles/PMC6760893/.
21. ICRP, *Report on the Task Group on Reference Man*, 1975.
22. Marcia Angell, *The Truth About the Drug Companies* (New York: Random House, 2005).
23. Naziba Sheikh, 'Why South Asian genes remember famine', Scientia News, 23 January 2025. Available at: https://www.scientianews.org/articles/genetics/why-south-asian-genes-remember-famine.
24. Sahih Muslim, 2052.
25. Angela M. Leung, Lewis E. Braverman and Elizabeth N. Pearce, 'History of U.S. Iodine Fortification and Supplementation', *Nutrients*, Vol. 4, 2012, pp. 1740–1746. Available at: https://files.givewell.org/files/DWDA%202009/Interventions/Iodine/Leung%2C%20Braverman%20and%20Pearce%202012.pdf.

26. Michael B. Zimmermann, et al., 'Increasing the iodine concentration in the Swiss iodized salt program markedly improved iodine status in pregnant women and children: a 5-y prospective national study', *American Journal of Clinical Nutrition*, Vol. 82(2), 2005, pp. 388–392. Available at: https://www.researchgate.net/publication/7672275.
27. Grand View Research, *Thyroid Support Supplements Market (2025–2033)*, 2025.
28. Béatrice S. Y. Choi, et al., 'Feeding diversified protein sources exacerbates hepatic insulin resistance via increased gut microbial branched-chain fatty acids and mTORC1 signaling in obese mice', *Nature Communications*, Vol. 12, 2021. Available at: https://www.nature.com/articles/s41467-021-23782-w.
29. Markham Heid, 'Experts Say Lobbying Skewed the U.S. Dietary Guidelines', *Time*, 8 January 2016. Available at: https://time.com/4130043/lobbying-politics-dietary-guidelines/.
30. Union of Concerned Scientists, *Delivering on the Dietary Guidelines*, 2019.
31. Ibid.
32. Palak Sanjeev Singhal, et al., 'Symptomatic Relief through Ayurveda Treatment in the Patient of Interstitial Lung Disease', *Journal of Ayurveda*, Vol. 17(3), 2023, pp. 266–272. Available at: https://www.ovid.com/journals/joay/fulltext/10.4103/joa.joa_174_22~symptomatic-relief-through-ayurveda-treatment-in-the-patient.
33. Charles Harding, et al., 'The daily, weekly, and seasonal cycles of body temperature analyzed at large scale', *Chronobiology International*, Vol. 36(12), 2019, pp. 1646–1657. Available at: https://pubmed.ncbi.nlm.nih.gov/31530024/.
34. Xiao-Gang Yuan, et al., 'Seasonal changes in gastric mucosal factors associated with peptic ulcer bleeding', *Experimental and Therapeutic Medicine*, Vol. 9(1), 2014, pp. 125–130. Available at: https://pmc.ncbi.nlm.nih.gov/articles/PMC4247295/.
35. Niranjan Raja, Hemachandar Radhakrishnan and Sivasankar Masilamani, 'Oxalate Nephropathy: A Case Report of Acute Kidney Injury Due to Juice Diet', *Cureus*, Vol. 15(12), 2023. Available at: https://pubmed.ncbi.nlm.nih.gov/38283477/.
36. Swetha Makkapati, Vivette D. D'Agati and Leah Balsam, '"Green Smoothie Cleanse" Causing Acute Oxalate Nephropathy', *American Journal of Kidney Diseases*, Vol. 71(2), 2023, pp. 281–286. Available at: https://pubmed.ncbi.nlm.nih.gov/29203127/.
37. Yu Zhang, et al., 'Porcine gut microbiota in mediating host metabolic adaptation to cold stress', *NPJ Biofilms and Microbiomes*, Vol. 8(1),

2022. Available at: https://pubmed.ncbi.nlm.nih.gov/35383199/.

38. Kelsey E. Huus and Ruth E. Ley, 'Blowing Hot and Cold: Body Temperature and the Microbiome', *mSystems*, 2021. Available at: https://journals.asm.org/doi/full/10.1128/msystems.00707-21.
39. Ajaikumar B. Kunnumakkara, et al., 'Role of Turmeric and Curcumin in Prevention and Treatment of Chronic Diseases: Lessons Learned from Clinical Trials', *ACS Pharmacology & Translational Science*, Vol. 6(4), 2023, pp. 447–518. Available at: https://pmc.ncbi.nlm.nih.gov/articles/PMC10111629/.
40. Canadian Foundation for Dietetic Research, *Functional Foods for Healthy Aging*, 2012.
41. Adeleh Sahebnasagh, et al., 'Therapeutic effects of crocin in alleviating diabetic neuropathy: a preliminary randomized triple-blind placebo-controlled trial', *Journal of Pharmaceutical Health Care and Sciences*, Vol. 11, 2025. Available at: https://link.springer.com/article/10.1186/s40780-025-00484-9.
42. Jose Lara, et al., 'Effects of inorganic nitrate and beetroot supplementation on endothelial function: a systematic review and meta-analysis', *European Journal of Nutrition*, Vol. 55(2), 2016, pp. 451–459. Available at: https://pubmed.ncbi.nlm.nih.gov/25764393/.
43. Pam Harrison, 'Beetroot Juice Lowers Blood Pressure in Hypertensives', Medscape, 2 December 2014. Available at: https://www.medscape.com/viewarticle/835666.
44. A. Patrician and E. Schagatay, 'Dietary nitrate enhances arterial oxygen saturation after dynamic apnea', *Scandinavian Journal of Medicine & Science in Sports*, Vol. 27(6), 2017, pp. 622–626. Available at: https://pubmed.ncbi.nlm.nih.gov/27037996/.
45. K. Honma, et al., 'Seasonal variation in the human circadian rhythm: dissociation between sleep and temperature rhythm', *American Journal of Physiology*, Vol. 262, 1992. Available at: https://pubmed.ncbi.nlm.nih.gov/1590482/.
46. Kyoko Fujihira, et al., 'Factors explaining seasonal variation in energy intake: a review', *Frontiers in Nutrition*, Vol. 10, 2023. Available at: https://pmc.ncbi.nlm.nih.gov/articles/PMC10400769.
47. H. Qui, et al., 'Influence of season on some skin properties: Winter vs. summer, as experienced by 354 Shanghaiese women of various ages', *International Journal of Cosmetic Science*, Vol. 33(4), 2011, pp. 377–383. Available at: https://www.researchgate.net/publication/50303235_Influence_of_season_on_some_skin_properties_Winter_vs_summer_as_experienced_by_354_Shanghaiese_women_of_various_ages.

48. Peter Chapman, *Bananas: How the United Fruit Company Shaped the World* (Edinburgh: Canongate, 2007).
49. 'What makes superfoods so super?' (Editorial), UC Davis. Available at: https://www.ucdavis.edu/food/news/what-makes-superfood-so-super#:~:text=The%20original%20superfood%E2%80%8B%E2%80%8B&text=The%20origin%20of%20the%20term,of%20cheap%2C%20easily%20digestible%20nutrition.
50. Fatemeh Sadat Hasheminasab, et al., 'Efficacy of the barley-based remedy, a Persian medicine formula, in coronavirus disease 2019 (COVID-19) hospitalized patients: An open-labeled randomized controlled trial', *Advances in Integrative Medicine*, Vol. 9(3), 2022, pp. 185–190. Available at: https://pmc.ncbi.nlm.nih.gov/articles/PMC9020837/.
51. Melissa Bailey, 'Sugar Industry Secretly Paid for Favorable Harvard Research', *Scientific American*, 13 September 2016. Available at: https://www.scientificamerican.com/article/sugar-industry-secretly-paid-for-favorable-harvard-research/.
52. Cristin E. Kearns, Laura A. Schmidt and Stanton A. Glantz, 'Sugar Industry and Coronary Heart Disease Research', *JAMA Internal Medicine*, Vol. 176(11), 2016, pp. 1680–1685. Available at: https://jamanetwork.com/journals/jamainternalmedicine/article-abstract/2548255.
53. Malene Lopez Kristensen, Palle Mark Christensen and Jesper Hallas, 'The effect of statins on average survival in randomised trials, an analysis of end point postponement', *BMJ Open*, Vol. 5(9), 2015. Available at: https://pubmed.ncbi.nlm.nih.gov/26408281/.
54. Morten Rix Hansen, et al., 'Postponement of Death by Statin Use: a Systematic Review and Meta-analysis of Randomized Clinical Trials', *Journal of General Internal Medicine*, Vol. 34(8), 2019, pp. 1607–1614. Available at: https://pubmed.ncbi.nlm.nih.gov/31073857/.
55. James J. Yang, 'Brain insulin resistance and the therapeutic value of insulin and insulin-sensitizing drugs in Alzheimer's disease neuropathology', *Acta Neurologica Belgica*, Vol. 122(5), 2022, pp. 1135–1142. Available at: https://pubmed.ncbi.nlm.nih.gov/35482277/.
56. Mithun Chandra Konar, et al., 'Effect of Virgin Coconut Oil Application on the Skin of Preterm Newborns: A Randomized Controlled Trial', *Annals of Tropical Paediatrics*, Vol. 66(2), 2022, pp. 129–135. Available at: https://pubmed.ncbi.nlm.nih.gov/31257430/.
57. Ibid.
58. Kriti Solanki, et al., 'Transcutaneous absorption of topically massaged oil in neonates', *Indian Pediatrics*, Vol. 42(10), 2005, pp. 998–1005.

Available at: https://pubmed.ncbi.nlm.nih.gov/16269830/.

59. Jess G. Fiedorowicz and William G. Haynes, 'Cholesterol, mood, and vascular health: Untangling the relationship', *Current Psychiatry Reports*, Vol. 9(7), 2010. Available at: https://pmc.ncbi.nlm.nih.gov/articles/PMC4215473.
60. Amir Faghihi, Mohammad Ebrahim Zohalinezhad and Majid Najafi Kalyani, 'Comparison of the Effects of Abdominal Massage and Oral Administration of Sweet Almond Oil on Constipation and Quality of Life among Elderly Individuals: A Single-Blind Clinical Trial', *BioMed Research International*, 2022. Available at: https://pmc.ncbi.nlm.nih.gov/articles/PMC9239810/.
61. Pedro Fong, et al., 'In silico prediction of prostaglandin D2 synthase inhibitors from herbal constituents for the treatment of hair loss', *Journal of Ethnopharmacology*, Vol. 175, 2015, pp. 470–480. Available at: https://pubmed.ncbi.nlm.nih.gov/26456343/.
62. Venkataram Mysore and Arpita Arghya, 'Hair Oils: Indigenous Knowledge Revisited', *International Journal of Trichology*, Vol. 14(3), 2022, pp. 84–90. Available at: https://pmc.ncbi.nlm.nih.gov/articles/PMC9231528/.
63. Ibid.
64. Yunes Panahi, et al., 'Rosemary oil vs minoxidil 2% for the treatment of androgenetic alopecia: a randomized comparative trial', *Skinmed*, Vol. 13(1), 2015, pp. 15–21. Available at: https://pubmed.ncbi.nlm.nih.gov/25842469/.
65. Ayad Mohammed Salem, et al., 'Effect of Nigella sativa supplementation on lung function and inflammatory mediators in partly controlled asthma: a randomized controlled trial', *Annals of Saudi Medicine*, Vol. 37(1), 2017, pp. 64–71. Available at: https://pmc.ncbi.nlm.nih.gov/articles/PMC6148976/.
66. Redhwan Ahmed Al-Naggar, et al., 'The Effects of Consuming Almonds and Almond Oil on Blood Lipids', *Asian Journal of Pharmaceutical Research and Health Care*, Vol. 15(1), 2023, pp. 1–10. Available at: https://journals.lww.com/ajpr/fulltext/2023/15010/.
67. Young Jun Kim, et al., 'Effect of herbal extracts on peripheral nerve regeneration after microsurgery of the sciatic nerve in rats', *BMC Complementary Medicine and Therapies*, Vol. 21, 2021. Available at: https://pmc.ncbi.nlm.nih.gov/articles/PMC8178854/.
68. Gottfried Novacek, 'Gender and gallstone disease', *Wiener Medizinische Wochenschrift*, Vol. 156(19–20), 2006, pp. 527–533. Available at: https://pubmed.ncbi.nlm.nih.gov/17103289/.
69. The Quran 31:14.